ADVANCED
S RF FITNESS

ADVANCED SURF FITNESS

FOR HIGH PERFORMANCE SURFING

LEE STANBURY

Advanced Surf Fitness for High Performance Surfing
ISBN 978-0-9567893-9-6

Printed and bound: Great Wall Printing, Hong Kong
Published by Orca Publications Limited, Berry Road Studios, Berry Road, Newquay, TR7 1AT, United Kingdom.
www.orcasurf.co.uk • +44 (0) 1637 878074

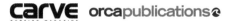

This book wouldn't have been possible without the help and support of the following people

MODELS/SURFERS Ben Skinner, Lee Bartlett
DESIGN David Alcock, Alistair Marshall
PHOTOGRAPHY Roger Sharp, Mike Searle
SURF PHOTOGRAPHY Roger Sharp, Mike Searle, Will Bailey, Mickey Smith
EDITORIAL CONSULTANT Steve England
PRODUCTION Louise Searle
PROOFREADERS Alex Hapgood, Hayley Spurway

DISCLAIMER: Before undertaking any course of fitness it is advisable to consult your doctor or physician. Whilst every effort has been made by the author and publishers to ensure that the information contained in this guide is accurate and up to date, they have neither the liability nor the responsibility for any loss, damage, death or injury arising from the information contained in this book.

COVER: Michel Bourez, Tahiti. **PHOTO:** Russell Ord

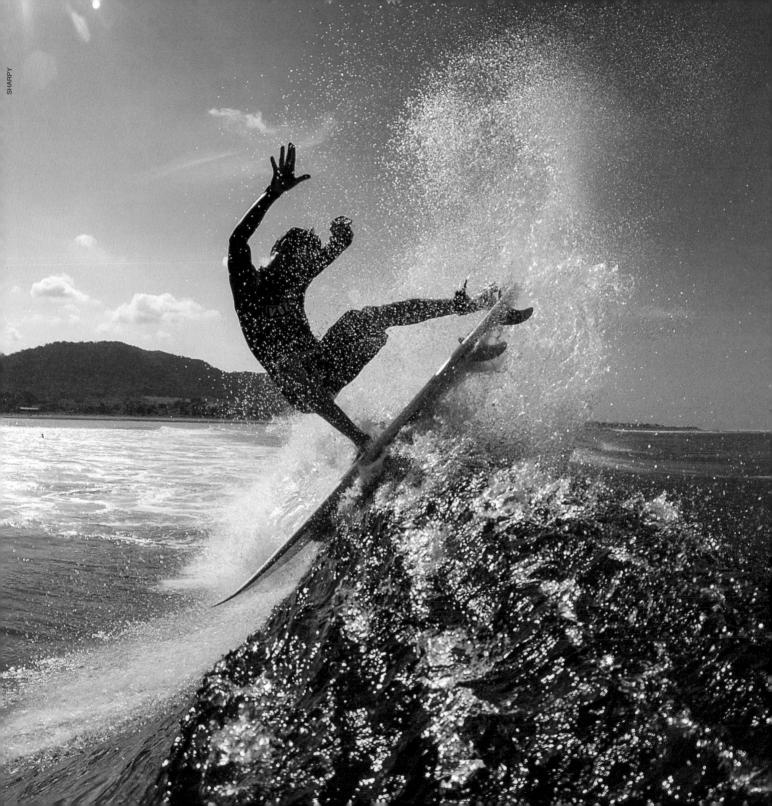

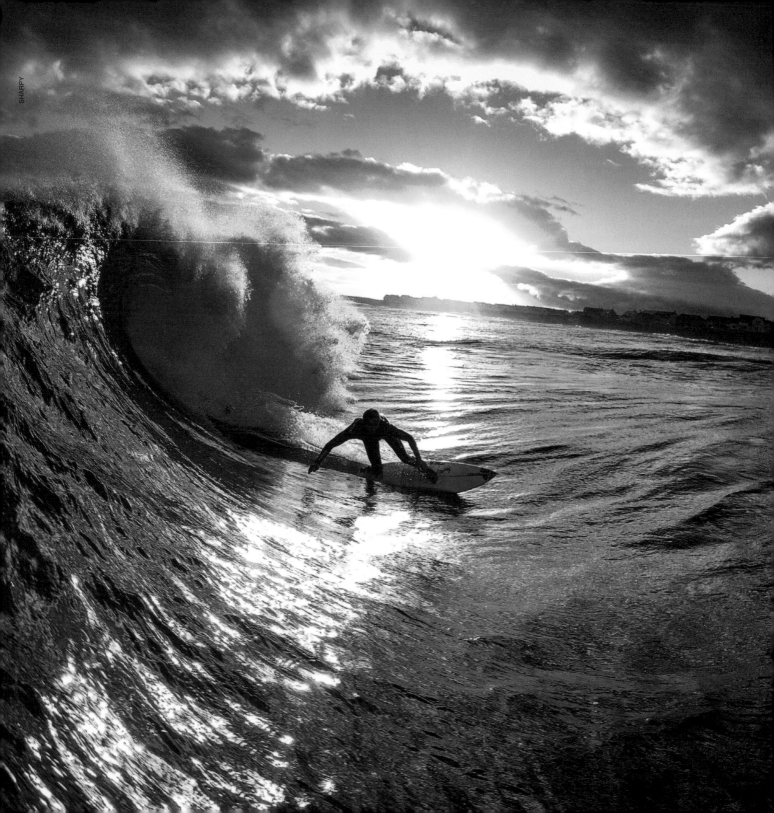

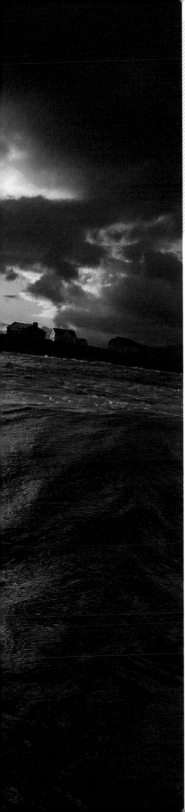

CONTENTS

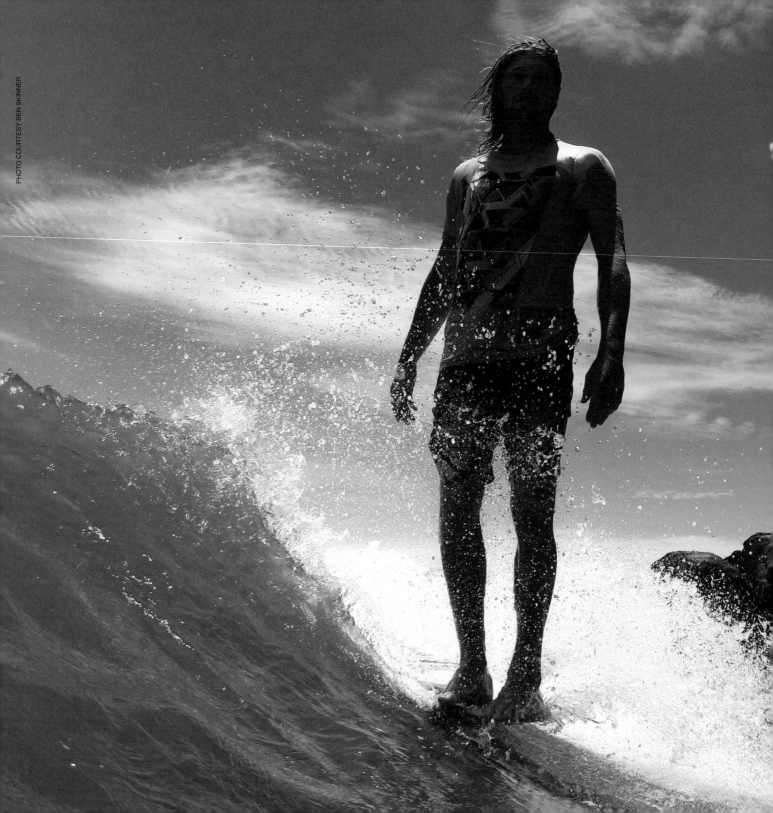

FOREWORD

By **BEN SKINNER** – 11 times European Longboard Champion

Surfing is a tough sport and it takes lot of effort to be on top of your game. In the past surfers mainly got away with just being in the water as much as possible – which was, and still is, great – but with the rise in performance levels and the amount of people in the water, most surfers now realise that it takes a lot of work if you are going to surf your best. The development of sports sciences and surf specific exercise are now being applied by surfers from all over the world, of all abilities, so that they can surf better. Elite surfers now realise a fitness coach is a necessary member of their team and fitness programmes – not only help them compete or ride bigger waves, but also help to prevent the injuries that go along with high performance surfing.

Being in peak fitness has helped me to achieve my goals of winning contests, surfing bigger waves and generally getting tubed as much as possible! The exercises we demonstrate in this book are the exercises I do on a regular basis, week in, week out. They have helped me to get fitter, stronger, more flexible and more confident so that, when it comes down to the wire, either in big waves or during a final, I can give it my all.

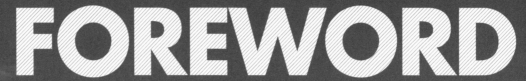

RICHARD DAVIES

There's no easy way around getting fit for surfing, you just have to man up and put the graft in, but it pays off in the end...

Good luck and stick with it!

– Ben

INTRO

By LEE STANBURY

Introduction to Surf Fitness and Performance

Surfing performance has moved upwards in a big way over the last 20 years. What was a lifestyle has become more professional with focus on diet, training and performance. Surfing movements have also improved massively and are more dynamic, explosive and now ever more airborne!

Be under no illusion: surfing is a physically challenging sport and todays manoeuvres can be highly demanding. Your surfing performance is governed by one thing and one thing alone and that is **your** body.

Your strength and fitness will determine how well you can perform, from paddling out, to catching waves amongst a crowd, increasing your confidence, pushing your limits in larger surf, as well as your surfing on the actual waves themselves.

Many surfers across the globe now see the benefits of land based surf fitness training for boosting their performance on the water. The list of additional training types is endless, but to be more specific you need to take a good look at your own performance. Do you lack paddle power? Are your cutbacks sluggish? Do you lack leg strength or is your stamina low? Maybe you think you lack the edge that other surfers always seem to have over you? Some surfers are not as lucky as others and may not get in the water that often, if this is the case then it's all the more reason to work hard on land so that when you do get in the water you are good to go.

These factors should all be addressed when constructing a surf fitness programme that will improve your performance and take your enjoyment of surfing to new heights. This book breaks down surf fitness into handy components from general paddle fitness to big wave surfing, and from pop ups to airs, with great exercises and top tips to help you surf to your own full potential.

So what are you waiting for?

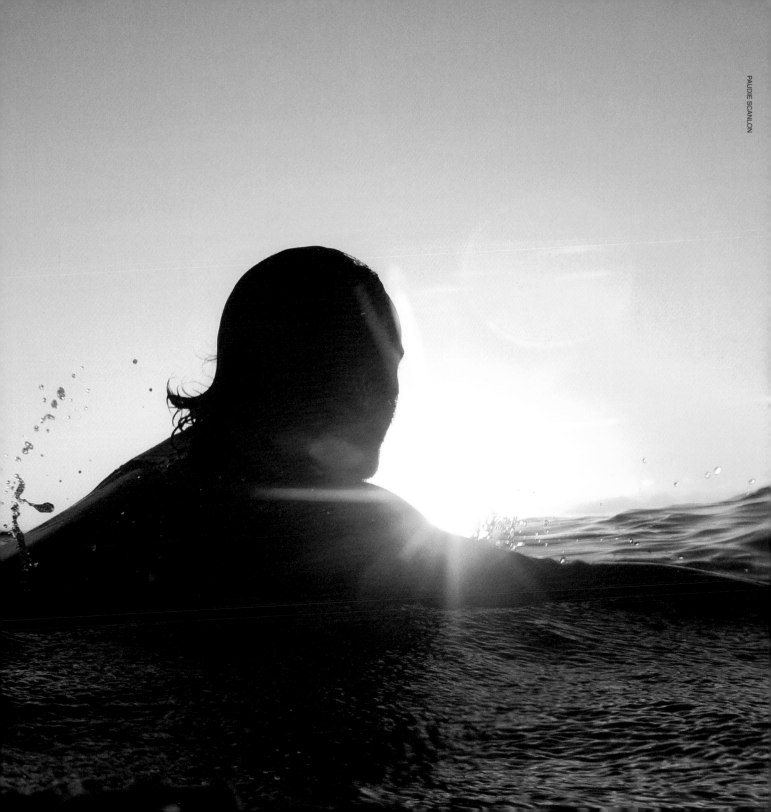

TRAINING KIT

Not so long ago a surfer just surfed. These days sports specific training and principles play an important role in improving performance. Regular surfers, landlocked surfers, surfing pros, young surfers and old surfers will all benefit from sports specific training that is tailored to them.

An abundance of kit is available nowadays, but here are some key pieces that are a must for any surfer:

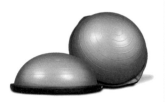

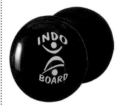

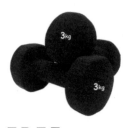

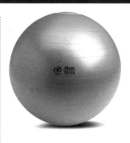

THE BOSU BALANCE TRAINER

The Bosu Balance trainer can be used both sides up, hence the name, "BOSU" (both sides utilised). This piece of equipment can be used for a huge range of training types, from core training to dynamic performance exercises.

THE INDO BOARD AND GIGANTE CUSHION

The Indo board has been around for many years and it has a wide range of uses. Now with the introduction of the Gigante cushion, the list of uses for the surfer is even more extensive.

FREE WEIGHTS

The physiological adoptions often associated with strength training include increases in muscle mass, bone mass and connective tissue thickness, with associated increases in muscle strength and endurance. All of these can be highly useful to a surfer, and strength for surfing movements can be gained by resistance training tailored specifically to the needs of the surfer.

THE SWISS BALL

The Swiss Ball is well know within the global surfing community as it is highly versatile and can be transported easily. Its uses run far and wide, from core strength training to surfing flexibility sessions. Many surfers use them on a regular basis to boost their surfing performance.

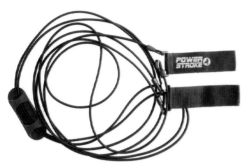

POWERSTROKE CORDS

PowerStroke Cords allow the surfer to go through specific paddle movements and build paddle strength. Take time to adjust the Power Stroke Bungee Cord's tension. You will need short practice sessions to really feel the benefits to your paddle power. You may need to practice general paddle power movements to find a good position that works best for you when using the Power Stroke Bungee Cord.

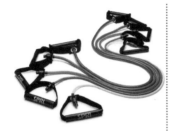

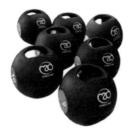

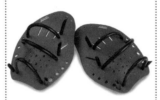

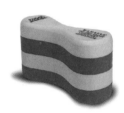

RESISTANCE BANDS

There are many types of these available – shorter cords will help isolate muscle groups which can improve a specific area.

MEDICINE BALLS

Medicine balls (also known as a fitness ball) are highly versatile weighted balls used effectively in plyometric weight training to increase explosive power in athletes in all sports.

HAND PADDLES

Hand paddles enhance the swimmer's feel of the "catch" – the phase prior to the pull, where the hand turns from a streamlined position to grasp the water and begin the pull. If the hand catches or pulls at an incorrect angle, the increased resistance afforded by the hand paddle will exacerbate the resulting twisting moment, making the defect clearer to the swimmer.

PULL-BUOY

Boost your upper body surfing power with swim pull sets. You simply place the buoys between your thighs and hold them there as you swim. This helps you keep your legs as motionless as possible, to concentrate on strengthening your upper body.

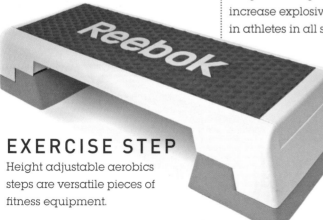

EXERCISE STEP

Height adjustable aerobics steps are versatile pieces of fitness equipment.

SHARPY

"IT'S ALL ABOUT WHERE YOUR MIND'S AT."

– KELLY SLATER

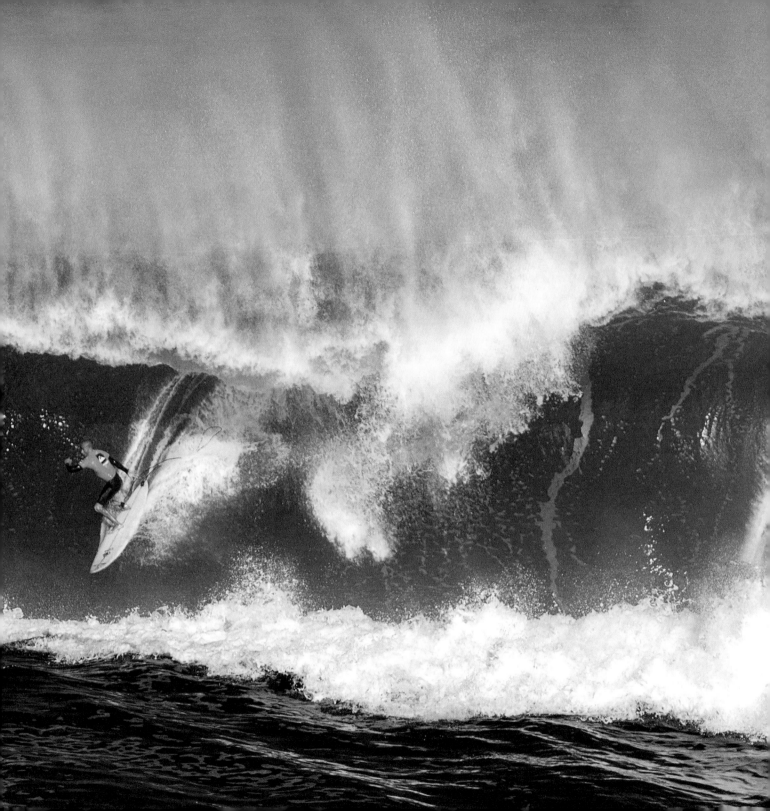

PRE-SURF WARM UP

There will always be that overwhelming temptation to run down the beach, straight into the surf and paddle out... But a basic mobility routine will only take 5-6 minutes and may mean the difference between a month off with an injury or injury free surfing with improved performance!

For a really great mobility warm up it is important to go through all the movements that you will use out in the water; aim for every body part with a little extra focus on back, hips and shoulders.

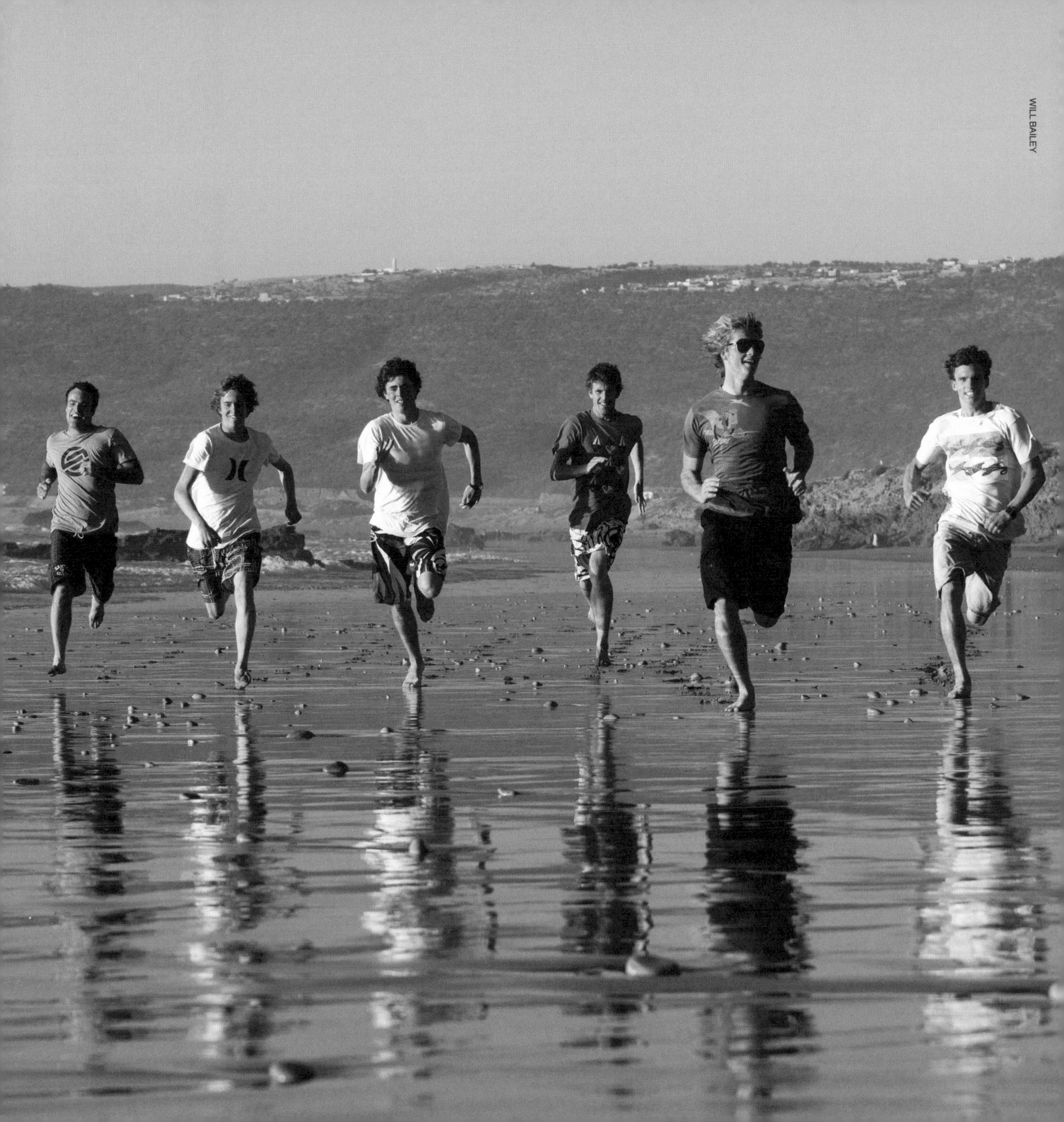

WILL BAILEY

THE BEST SURFING WARM UP

WHY ARE WE WARMING UP?

AS YOU PREPARE YOUR BODY TO SURF IT'S IMPORTANT TO THINK ABOUT JUST WHAT YOU ARE WARMING UP: LIGAMENTS, TENDONS AND MUSCLES SENDING RICH OXYGENATED BLOOD TO THE VITAL AREAS SO THAT YOUR PADDLE OUT (AND YOUR FIRST FEW WAVES) ARE DONE WITH THE LEAST AMOUNT OF EFFORT.

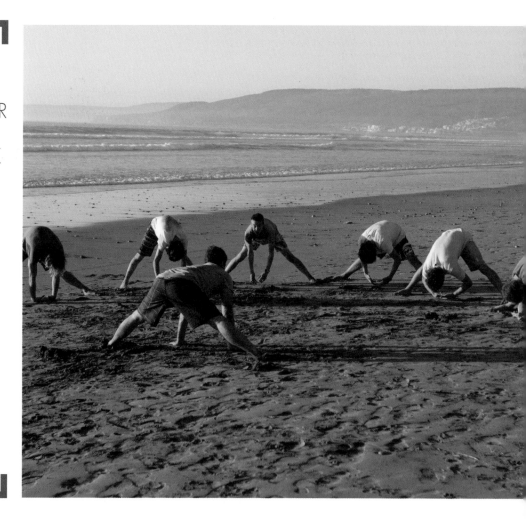

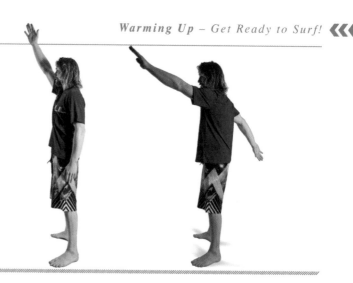

BASIC ARM SWINGS...

A simple but effective light exercise that will get you ready for a paddle out.

Standing with your feet hip width apart and facing forwards, with relaxed arms swing your left arm forwards 10 times before repeating on the other side, after this reverse the movement.

SLOW NECK ROTATIONS...

Warming up the neck with mobility can help prevent neck strains.

Slowly drop your chin downwards and rotate your neck in a clockwise movement. Do this 5 times to the left and then repeat 5 times to the right.

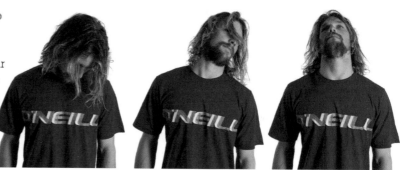

SHOULDER RETRACTIONS...

The muscles around the shoulder blades can be very complex. There's a lot going on in this area and it needs a good warm up.

Standing forwards again slowly raise your shoulders upwards and backwards lifting shoulders upwards to your ears; as you do these squeeze your shoulder blades together.

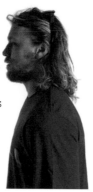
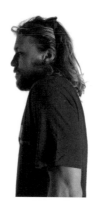
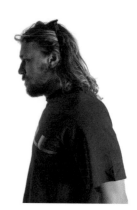

ROTATE AND DROP...

This is a great exercise for warming up the lower back, a key area during paddling movements.

With your feet a hip width apart start with your arms in the air, then swing your arms downwards towards your feet. Begin with the left side before repeating on the right. 10 times on each side.

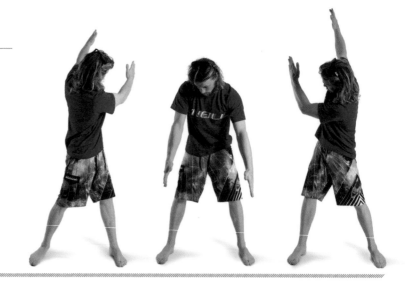

BENT OVER ARM SWINGS...

Again this is an area for major consideration, if you're keen to paddle out back faster, then this area of mobility is key.

Stand with your feet about a hip width apart with soft knees. Lean forwards and let your arms hang downwards, then swing your arms so that you reach backwards to slap your back. Repeat 10 times.

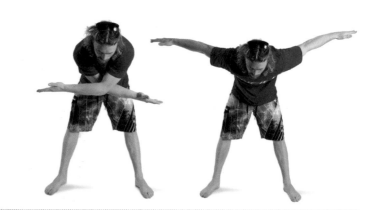

SPINAL ROTATIONS...

Just think of all the movements in surfing – the complexities of bio mechanics are massive and the spine (erectus spine) is a major muscle group.

Standing feet forwards arms out to the sides, slowly turn to the left as far as you can go, then repeat on the other side.

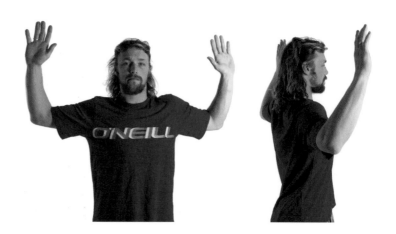

BACKWARD /FORWARDS LEG SWINGS...

Many surfers will at some point get a groin strain. This simple leg exercise can help in this area through warming up the hip flexors and preparing your body for that first pop up!

Relax your left leg and simply let it swing backwards and forwards 10 times before repeating on the other side. You may need the support of a partner for this.

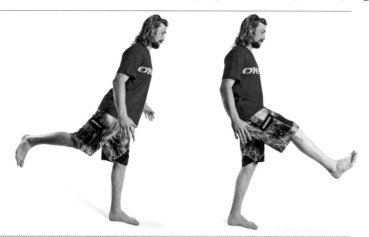

HIP ROTATIONS...

Wake up the hip area further which will also help with your first few pop ups.

Stand facing forwards, slowly bring your knee upwards to the left then turn your knee outwards to the side before returning it to the starting position.

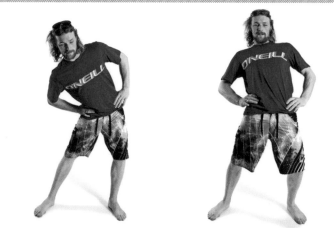

LEG SWING CROSS OVER...

This is also a great exercise for warming up hip flexors and preparing for pop ups.

Relax and swing your leg across your body line to the left before swinging back to the starting position. Do this 10 times before repeating on the other side. Again, you may need support for this.

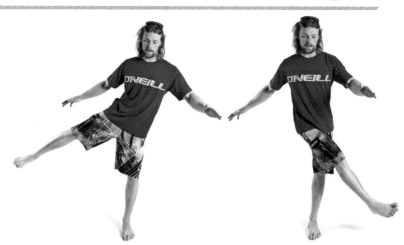

SIDE BENDS...

This nice mobility exercise will lightly warm up the latissimus dorsi muscles.

Stand with feet a hip width apart, arms in the air, then slowly bend over to the left side keeping your arms in the air. Maintain a good body alignment – repeat this 10 times on each side.

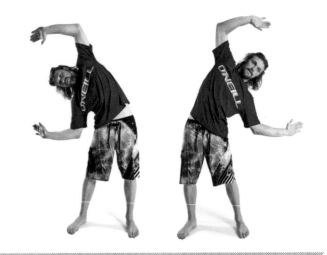

ANKLE ROTATIONS...

Good ankle flexibility plays a central role in moving your board around so warming up the ankle is key for those first few movements.

With hands on hips, point your toes to the floor and slowly rotate your foot clockwise. Do this 10 times before repeating the other way.

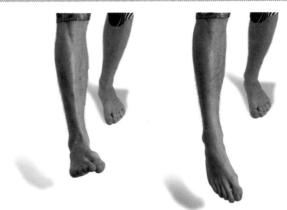

BASIC KNEE LIFTS...

A simple knee lift is a good way of warming up the knees, which is also going to aid with your first few waves.

Start with your foot on the ground and simply bring the knee upwards. Lift your knee up to your chest 8-10 times.

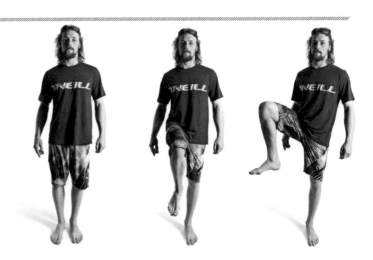

HAMSTRING STRETCH...

Start by sitting on the floor, legs outstretched, then slowly lean forwards, with arms extended. Once you reach the point of discomfort stop, hold for 10-15 seconds then move slowly back to the starting position.

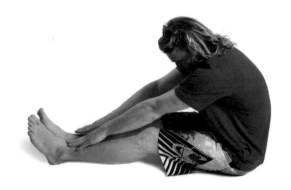

POP UP TO JUMPS...

Once you have this basic warm up in place you can have a go at more specific dynamic movements which mimic your surfing movements.

Simply jump upwards bringing one knee up towards your chest. Repeat 4 times on each leg.

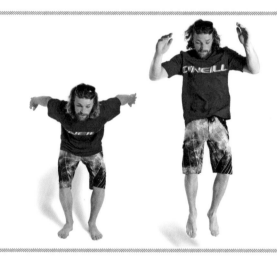

TATYANA VYC/SHUTTERSTOCK.COM

IMPORTANT TO REMEMBER

WHEN UNDERTAKING ANY PRE-EXERCISE MOBILITY MOVEMENTS, IT IS IMPORTANT TO USE A SMOOTH CONTROLLED MOTION. YOU SHOULD START WITH SMALL MOVEMENTS AND ONLY USE A LARGER RANGE OF MOVEMENT AS YOUR REPS PROGRESS.

ASSESSING YOUR SURF FITNESS

There are many tests available for assessing your surf fitness. Some can be pretty advanced but there are many that are also very simple and these can be a great asset if you're looking to improve your surfing and surf fitness.

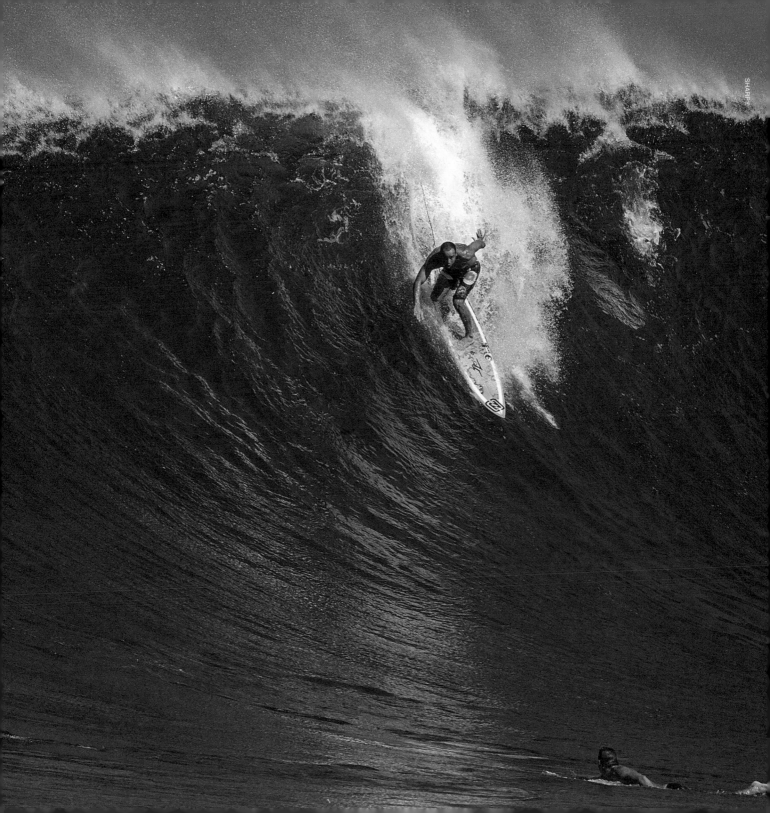

STRENGTHENING YOUR CORE

So much emphasis is put on "Core Training", whether it's for general fitness, rehabilitation or sport performance. Why? Because it's your body's foundation for movement, power, stabilization and protection... So, a poor core impedes your fitness, and can leave you wide open to injury. In surfing terms, a strong core enables you to improve your power, performance and stability, which will help you to both catch the wave of your life and ride it down the line with coordinated style!

THE FRONT PLANK TEST

TEST YOUR CORE STRENGTH

Position yourself so that your toes are on the ground and your elbows are directly below your shoulders, then raise yourself up keeping a straight line from your shoulders through to your ankles, so that your elbows and toes support your body.

Use your tummy muscles to maintain the position, keep your head in line with your spine and try not to stick your bottom in the air! Hold this position for as long as possible.

DATE	DURATION

Take note of the time. As the weeks pass and your core strength improves there should be vast improvements in the length of time you can hold a front plank.

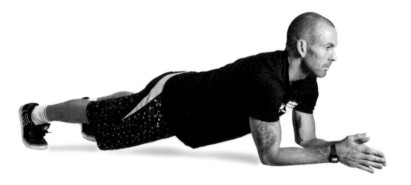

HOW STRONG IS YOUR CORE? WHAT IS CORE STRENGTH?

The core muscles include not only those in your abdominals and back, but also muscles in your pelvic floor and hips. Many of your core muscles can't be seen because they're buried underneath other muscles. The transverse abdominals, for example, hide underneath your rectus abdominals and encase the whole area below the belly button. While the rectus abdominals are sitting on top looking good, the transverse abdominals are working hard – especially during surfing movements.

TESTING EXPLOSIVE POWER

VERTICAL JUMP TEST

This test is designed to test your explosive leg power. For a surfer this can be important because as any surf session progresses and tiredness sets in, explosive leg power diminishes.

All you need is a high wall. Start the test by standing side on to the wall and make a note of how high you can reach without jumping. This is your standing reach height. Then stand slightly away from the wall and, using both arms to aid your upwards movement, touch the wall at the highest point of your jump.

Make a note of where you touched the wall, then make a measurement of the distance between the standing reach height and the jump height and this is your result. Try the test every 6-8 weeks.

DATE	HEIGHT

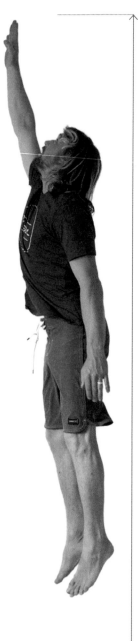

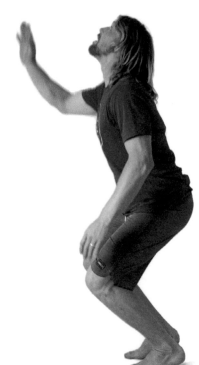

[BOOSTING YOUR LEG STRENGTH WILL IMPROVE YOUR STAMINA AND LENGTHEN YOUR SURF SESSIONS.]

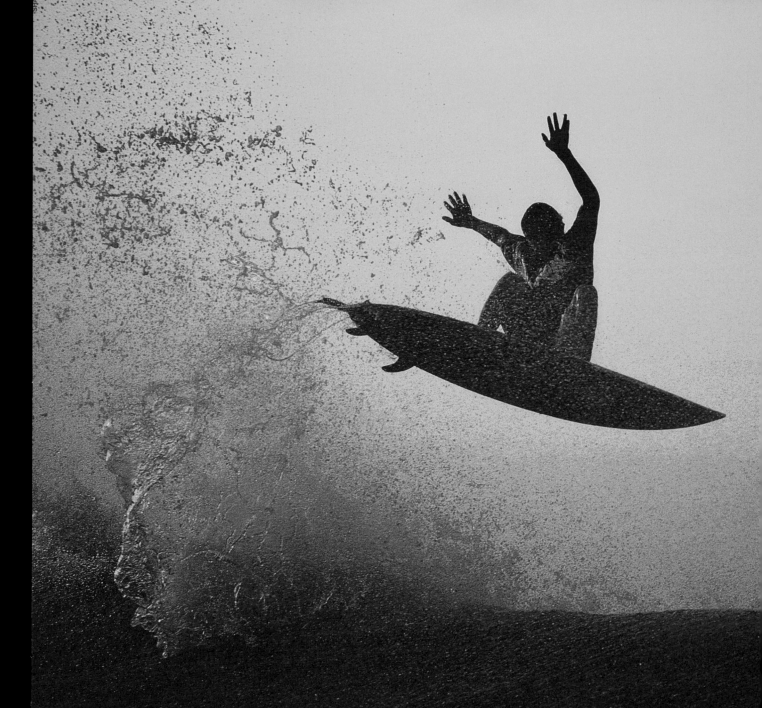

FLEXIBILITY TESTS
WHY TEST FLEXIBILITY FOR SURFING?

Flexibility tests can be used to:

Make assessments on your range of movement

Make general assessments on your muscle imbalances

Chart your flexibility progression as you train

THE SIT AND REACH TEST

The sit and reach test is very simple and can be a good guide for testing your flexibility in the lower back and hamstrings.

Before you start the test you will need a tape measure long enough so that it reaches from the middle knee area to just past your toes.

To begin the test sit down with your legs extended and your back up against the wall. Then run the tape measure from the knees down the middle of your legs just past your toes. Place one hand over the other then slowly reach forwards. Make a note of how far you can reach, repeat 3 times and record your distance.

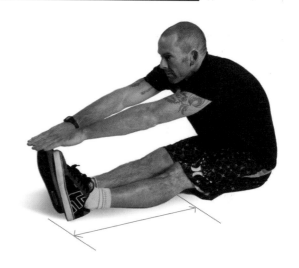

35 METRES SPRINT TEST

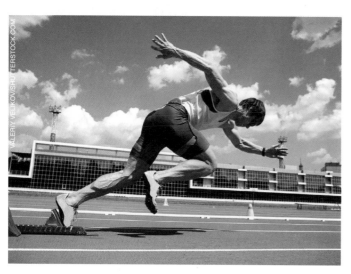

The objective of the sprint speed test is to assess the athlete's sprint acceleration. This test is best done with 2 people so the times are accurate.

To begin the test, warm up for 10 minutes. Mark out a flat 35 metre straight section to sprint along. The athlete conducts 3 x 35 metre sprints with a 5 minute recovery between each sprint. The assistant times the sprints and uses the fastest time to assess the athlete's performance.

Rating	Male	Female
Excellent	< 4.80	< 5.30
Good	4.80 - 5.09	5.30 - 5.59
Average	5.10 - 5.29	5.60 - 5.89
Fair	5.30 - 5.60	5.90 - 6.20
Poor	> 5.60	> 6.20

TRUNK ROTATION TEST

This is a great test for trunk flexibility, which is vital for the sharp dynamic movements that we use when surfing.

Start by marking a vertical line on the wall, then stand about an arm's length away from the wall with your feet a shoulder width apart and with your back to the wall directly in front of the line.

Extend your arms out directly in front of you so they are parallel to the floor, then slowly twist your trunk to your right and touch the wall behind you with your fingertips. Your arms should stay extended and parallel to the floor. You can turn your shoulders, hips and knees as long as your feet don't move.

Mark the position where your fingertips touched the wall. Measure the distance from the line. A point before the line is a negative score and a point after the line is a positive score.

Repeat for the left side and take the average of the two scores and use the table provided below to rate your score.

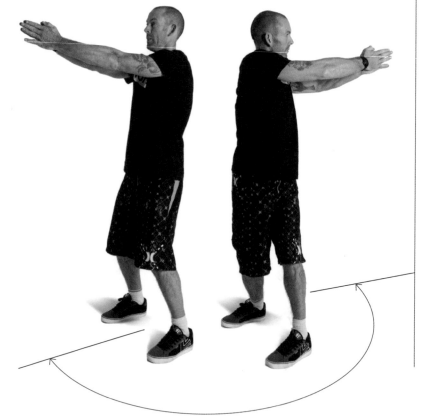

Trunk Rotation Test Evaluation Sheet

POOR- NEED WORK!	FAIR	GOOD	VERY GOOD!	EXCELLENT
-0CM	-5CM	-10CM	-15CM+	-20CM+

BASIC STRENGTH TEST

A BASIC PRESS UP TEST

Although this is a basic test it's a good way of testing your upper body strength as a press up brings into play many of the upper body muscle groups. Popping up demands upper body strength and the longer your surf session is the harder this upper body move will become.

Start the test in a press up position, then try as many press ups as possible in 1 minute. Record the number of press ups and repeat every 2 weeks.

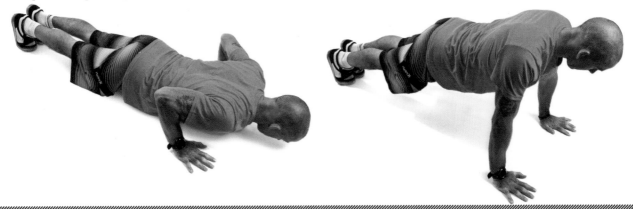

AEROBIC SWIMMING TEST

Testing aerobic fitness to gauge surfing paddle power can be tricky. This said, most surfers will know that if they've been finding it hard to paddle out or if stamina for catching waves dips halfway through a session, their aerobic endurance needs attention.

The Swim Time Trial
- Before starting the test mobility is a must so warm up properly for 6-8 minutes.
- Then swim as far as possible in 20 minutes.
- Record the distance (lengths) and repeat on a monthly basis
- To improve your results adopt a regular swim programme and notice the difference in your paddle power and aerobic fitness in a few weeks.

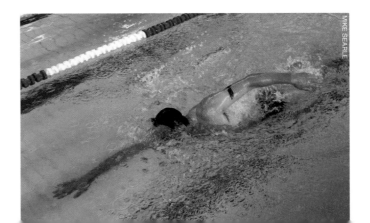

MIKE SEARLE

WHEN YOU FEEL LIKE QUITTING, THINK ABOUT WHY YOU STARTED

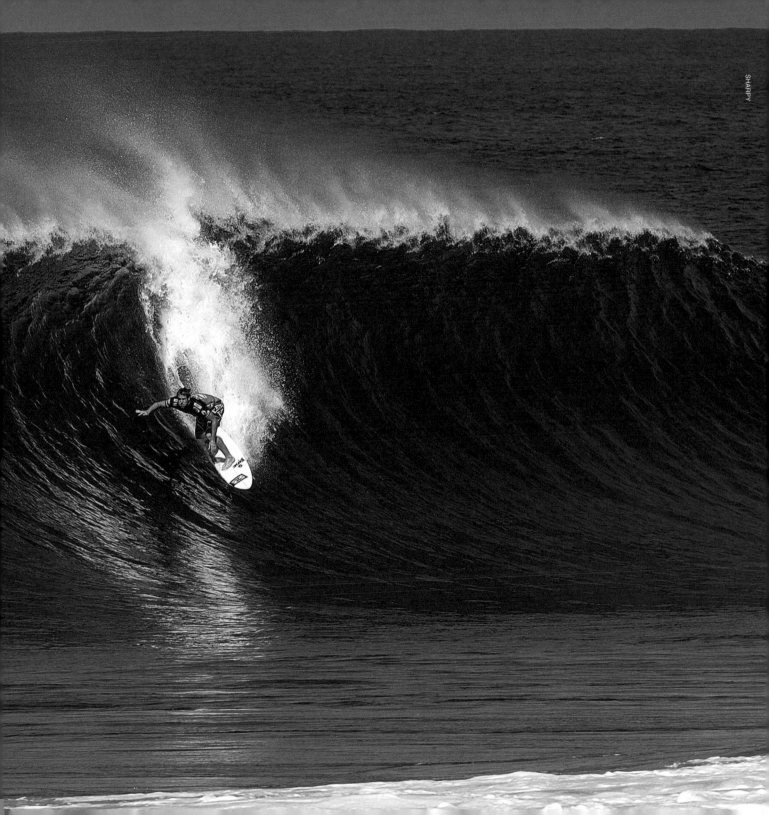

CO-ORDINATION AND BALANCE

Understanding your surfing movements and the muscle groups that drive those movements is the key to improving your surfing performance. For a surfing movement to be enhanced it first needs to be trained. Of course repetitive surfing movements out at your local break help, but there will always be factors that restrict progression. A poor day of waves, inconsistent swell patterns, lack of time – if we all had no other commitments other than to surf, or we had perfect waves every day we would all be better surfers and have less cause to keep fit on land.

Thankfully improvements in your dynamic surfing movements can be achieved from improving muscle coordination and balance.

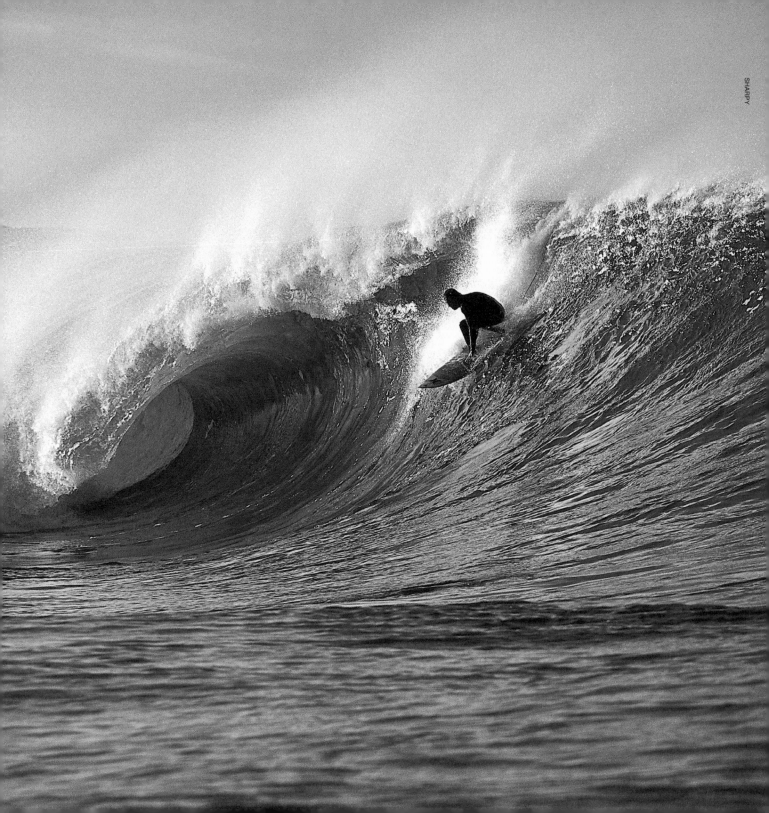

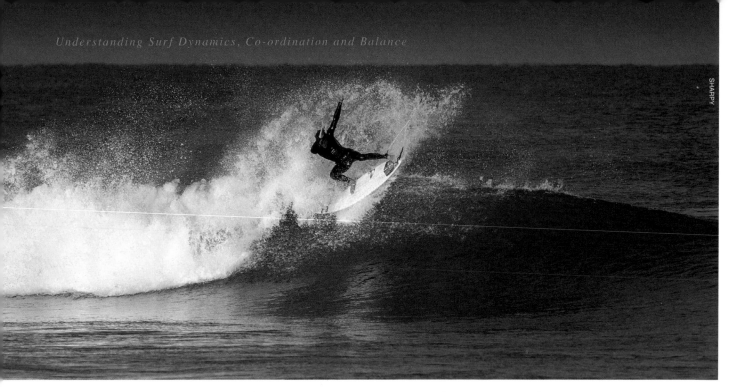

SHARPY

BALANCE TRAINING FOR IMPROVEMENTS IN DYNAMIC SURFING MOVEMENTS

Balance plays a key role in the development of surfing performance and enjoyment. There are many factors to take into account while developing sports balance and once you understand these factors development can take place at a faster pace.

LONG TERM ATHLETE DEVELOPMENT (LTAD) OF SURFING PERFORMANCE

As a surfer progresses with their general surfing movements, there are more demands placed on these movements. With surfing at any level there is always a new challenge to face, a new movement or a sharper movement. For any surfer wishing to improve their surfing technique it is important to understand the dynamics of sporting movements. This encourages a greater understanding of how it is possible to train for greater performance.

'Natural' surfing talent and progression often comes from simply learning to surf at a very young age. It is true that between the ages of one and eleven the human body's ability to learn a new skill like surfing is at its strongest as the young body develops its neuromuscular pathways.

The speed at which a surfer develops their dynamic movements may also be governed by muscle type. Slow twitch muscle fibres and fast twitch fibres have very different contractile and metabolic characteristics. For example, it is known that movement and quickness depends on which of the two an athlete is born with. A sprinter will have a high percentage of fast twitch fibres while a distance runners muscles will contain a higher percentage of slow twitch fibres.

Despite this, the fact is that movements for surfing quickness and performance can be trained, and it is possible to train these key surfing elements at any age. Although the longer a surfer is left in their natural state of development the harder it will be. So the saying "You can't teach an old dog new tricks" does become truer with time!

WHY SHOULD I USE BALANCE TRAINING FOR IMPROVEMENTS IN SURFING PERFORMANCE?

- Enhances co-ordination, balance, neuromuscular function and athletic movements.
- Develops and keeps sensory feedback systems sharp and well trained. Neuromuscular training increases movement efficiency regardless of activity.
- Helps to develop balance and stabilising strength that will result in improved posture and better endurance during surfing movements.
- Helps create a new sense of body awareness, position and movement confidence.

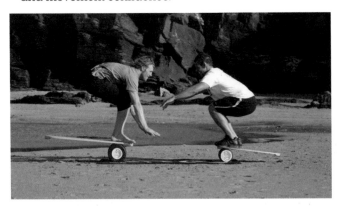

FUNCTIONAL BALANCE TRAINING AND SURFING MOVEMENTS

Balance and stabilisation training can be thought of as a position, or series of positions, that occur during surfing movements and are maintained when opposing forces equalise one another so that little or no movement occurs at the stabilised joint. This means that muscles on both sides of the joint contribute to stabilising via a co-contraction of agonist and antagonistic muscles.

Balance: Movement built upon this function represents an ability to stabilise and maintain a desired body position. Balance can be thought of as a correct or effective positioning of a body part or the entire body. This can be clearly seen during many surfing movements.

BASIC DYNAMIC EXERCISES FOR IMPROVEMENTS IN SURFING DYNAMICS AND COORDINATION

It is possible to improve your surfing dynamics, coordination and balance by training on the land.

An example to improve leg movements and coordination could be a basic jump and stick.

Start the exercise in a basic press up position, then explode forwards at speed with both legs, then stick in that spot and hold that position before repeating. In this way you can train your body to be more explosive. It is possible to build and develop speed, coordination and balance.

Even a basic jump and squat can build strength in this area. Start the exercise in the press up position, then bring both feet forwards at speed, tucking your knees upwards. From here jump up vertically then repeat, do the exercise 10 times then rest.

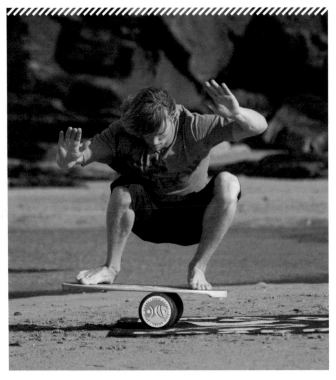

TRAINING FOR **COORDINATED** **SURFING MOVEMENTS**

There are many diverse movements in surfing which can sometimes take years to master. Repeating surfing movements in a land based programme and adding resistance like free weights or medicine balls can make a great difference to that movement.

An example could be a roundhouse cutback – a demanding movement but with the right training and exercise this can be improved and sharpened.

BALANCE SQUAT AND THROW OVER

For best results use an unstable balance training aid like the Indo board or Bosu Balance trainer, plus a medicine ball for added resistance to the move.

Start the move in a squat position, then extend upwards, bringing the ball over your shoulder to mimic a multi-directional movement, then repeat. Do this on both sides of the body.

During a roundhouse there are many demands on the body's ability to balance, and core strength can be tested to the max the sharper the movement gets.

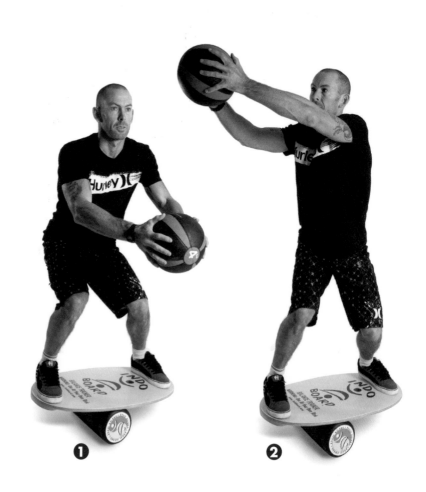

①   **②**

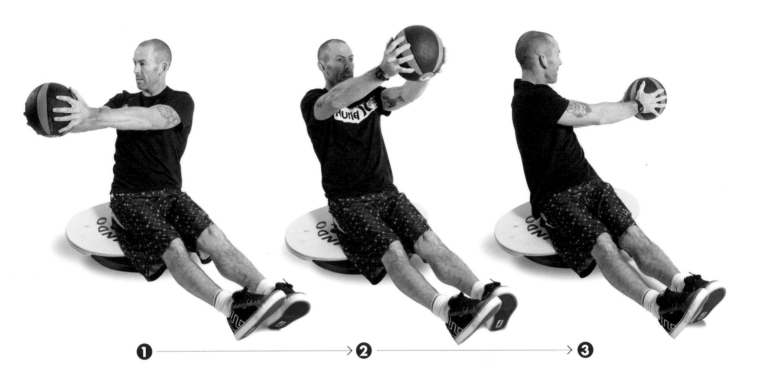

SEATED MEDICINE BALL TWIST

A cutback can also be improved by a seated medicine ball twist. This is based on a Russian twist and works the abdomen muscles, building explosiveness in the upper torso. Using the Gigante and Indo board increases the work done by the muscles.

Start with your feet together and the ball in both hands, with the ball resting on the floor just alongside your hips. Swing the ball from side to side keeping your body upright. The slower you move your arms from side to side, the harder the exercise becomes. Repeat the exercise, 10 times on each side before resting.

SEATED MEDICINE BALL THROWS

To make things harder, you can use a partner to throw the ball to. Throw the ball to a partner, they will then throw back to you repeating the exercise as before, 10 times on one side and 10 times on the other before resting.

THE BENEFITS OF STRENGTH TRAINING FOR SURFERS

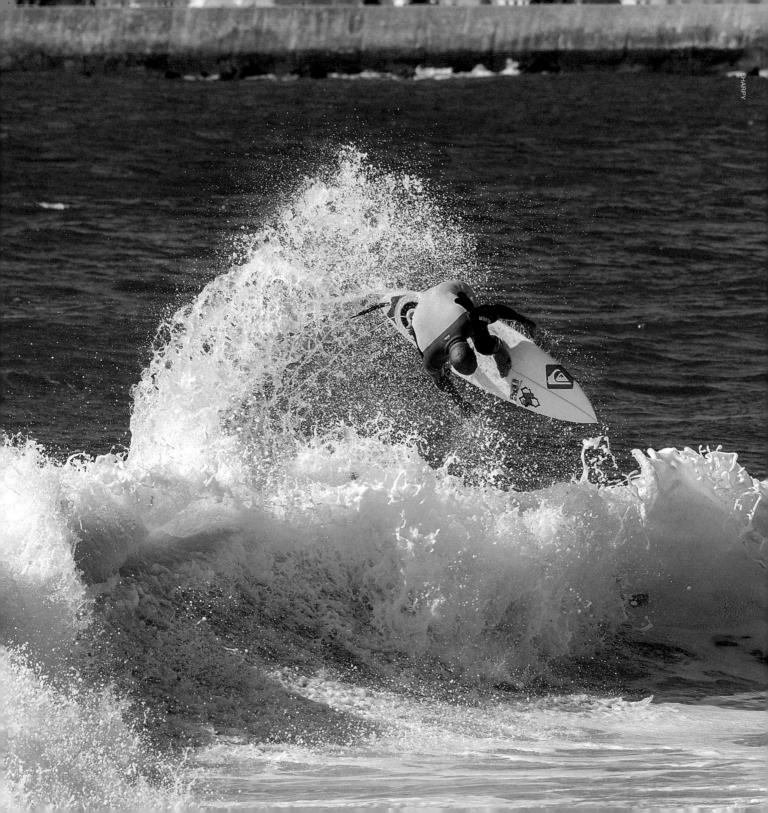

SHARPY

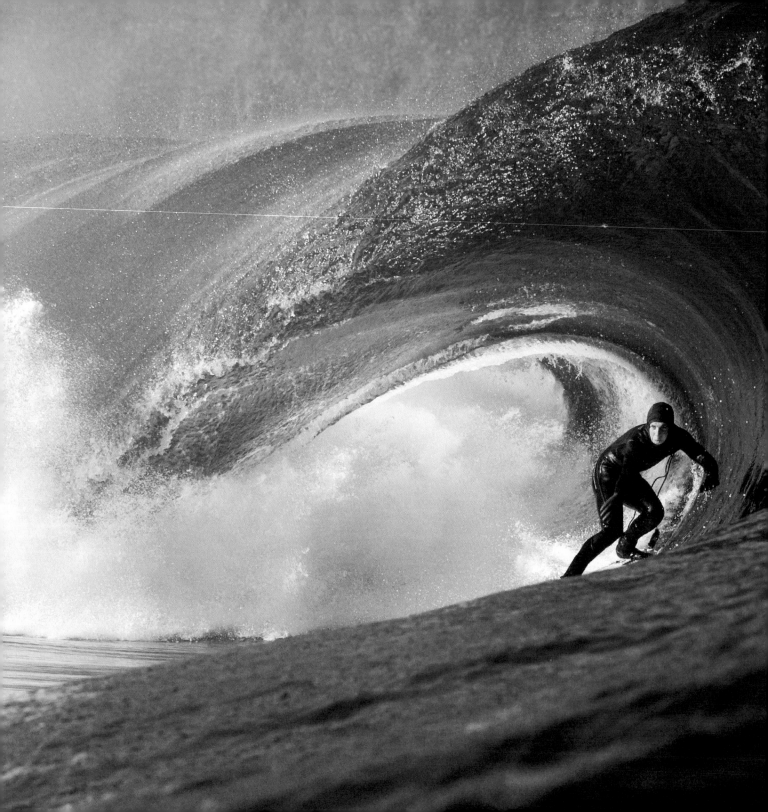

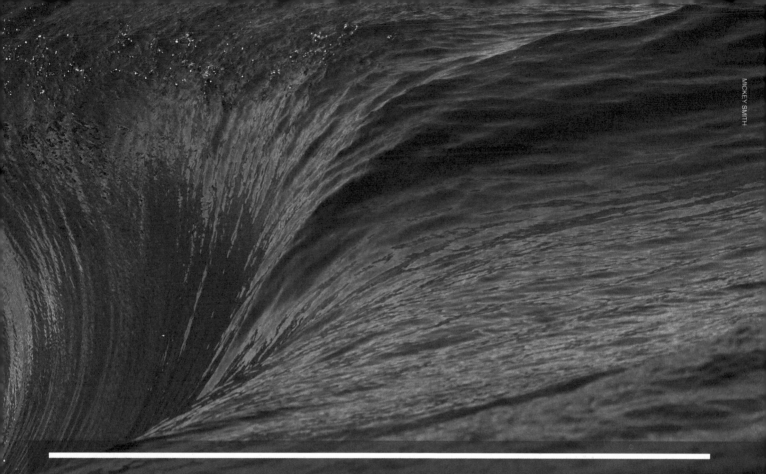

The physiological adaptations most often associated with strength training are increases in muscle mass, bone mass and connective tissue thickness, with associated increases in muscle strength and endurance. All of these are very relevant to a surfer.

Strength during surfing movements can be gained by resistance training, but not just any strength training will do. For example there are specific types of strength training for specific sports, and different types of training that offer different outcomes.

Strength training isn't just about lifting weights (although weight training can be highly beneficial to surfing strength), there are many more strength training types that can also be of great benefit.

The ability to generate strength is an essential component for success in many sports, and particularly in those involving explosive movements – such as surfing.

Key elements in strength training for surfers

With strength training to improve surfing performance, there are key areas to take into consideration. For 'true' strength gains to take place you need to look at just what surfing movements you are trying to strengthen and why, and the strength exercises must be functional for that move. For example, if your goal is to improve your upper body strength for improved paddle fitness, you wouldn't lift massive weights which could restrict your range of movement (ROM).

During surfing performance, endurance is a key factor. Paddling out plays a major part in surfing at whatever level you're at, and whatever size the surf is. For a surfer to use strength training to improve their paddle power, endurance strength training would be the key.

ELEMENTS OF
STRENGTH TRAINING

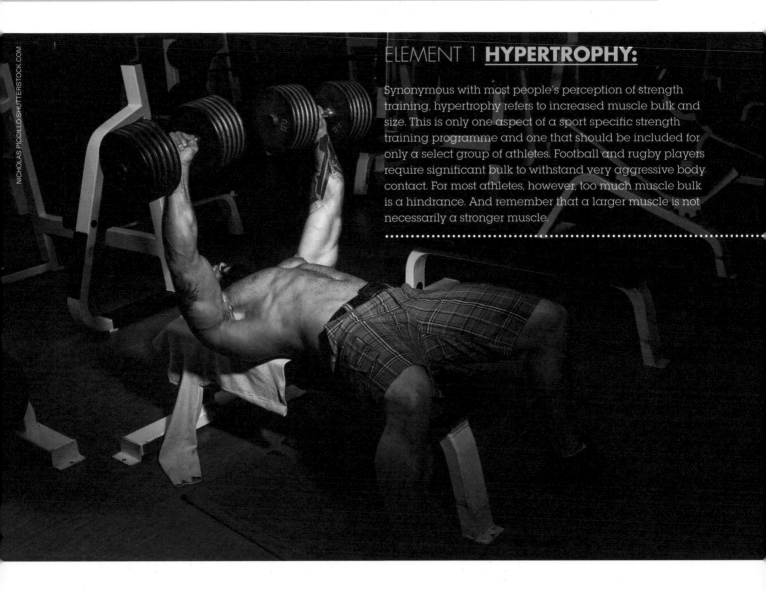

ELEMENT 1 **HYPERTROPHY:**

Synonymous with most people's perception of strength training, hypertrophy refers to increased muscle bulk and size. This is only one aspect of a sport specific strength training programme and one that should be included for only a select group of athletes. Football and rugby players require significant bulk to withstand very aggressive body contact. For most athletes, however, too much muscle bulk is a hindrance. And remember that a larger muscle is not necessarily a stronger muscle.

ELEMENT 2 **STRENGTH ENDURANCE:**

Strength endurance is defined as the ability to perform for long periods of time without, or with minimal decrease in output and muscle efficiency. Basically you can surf for longer with a minimal drop in performance. Or perform press ups for a long period with good technique. This could be defined for events such as distance running, cycling, swimming and long surf sessions, where strength endurance is a major factor.

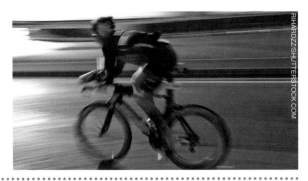

[STRENGTH ENDURANCE CAN BE DEVELOPED THROUGH 'OWN BODY WEIGHT' EXERCISES LIKE PULL UPS OR PRESS UPS, OR THE USE OF LOW WEIGHTS AND HIGH REPETITIONS. AGAIN IT IS IMPORTANT TO SAY THAT STRENGTH TRAINING FOR SURFERS SHOULD NOT RESTRICT SURFING MOVEMENTS AND THIS SHOULD BE TAKEN INTO ACCOUNT WHEN DESIGNING A SURF FITNESS PROGRAMME.]

ELEMENT 3 **EXPLOSIVE POWER:**

This is a key element when developing a strength programme for surfers. The dynamic movements are key to performance so any strength training should be aimed at this area as a priority.

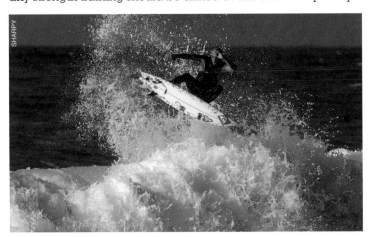

THE BENEFITS

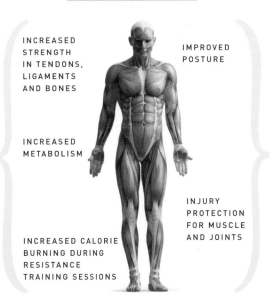

INCREASED STRENGTH IN TENDONS, LIGAMENTS AND BONES

IMPROVED POSTURE

INCREASED METABOLISM

INJURY PROTECTION FOR MUSCLE AND JOINTS

INCREASED CALORIE BURNING DURING RESISTANCE TRAINING SESSIONS

CLASSIFICATIONS OF STRENGTH

THE THREE CLASSIFICATIONS OF STRENGTH ARE:

Maximum strength - the greatest force that is possible in a single maximum contraction.

Elastic strength - the ability to overcome a resistance with a fast contraction.

Strength endurance - the ability to express force many times over (this is a key factor in surfing fitness and performance).

HOW DO WE GET STRONGER FOR SURFING USING WEIGHTS?

A muscle will only strengthen when forced to operate beyond its customary intensity (known as 'overload'). Overload can be progressed by increasing the:

Resistance. (for example the amount of weight lifted.)
Number of repetitions with a particular weight.
Number of sets in the exercise.

Gains in surfing strength can be achieved from using weights, but it is important to remember that the correct type of weight training must be done. A light to intermediate weight should be used and sets of a high rep count (15-30 upwards) should be done, as this will build strength endurance.

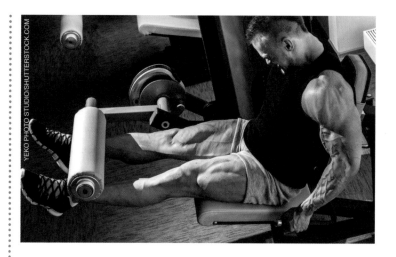

YEKO PHOTO STUDIO/SHUTTERSTOCK.COM

STRENGTH TRAINING TERMINOLOGY

Here are just a few terms used in strength training:

Strength: the amount of force a muscle can exert against a resistance.

Resistance: any force acting in opposition to a contraction.

Overload: progressive resistance beyond what is comfortable or moderately uncomfortable. Overload is dependent upon intensity, duration and frequency.

Set: number of repetitions done consecutively with no break between them.

Tempo: the speed with which an exercise is performed.

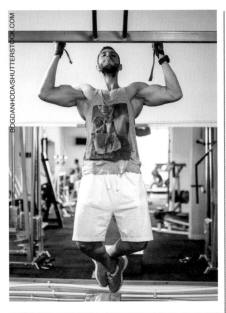

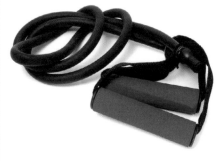

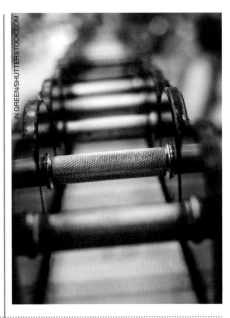

STRENGTH TRAINING WITH YOUR OWN BODY WEIGHT

Using your own body weight for gains in surfing strength can be highly beneficial, and there's no equipment needed.

During surfing movements there are many demands on the legs; even a basic bottom turn will demand strength and drive from the gluteus maximus (buttocks) for example.

RESISTANCE BANDS AND CORDS

In addition to your own body weight for strength training, another form of resistance and strength training can be done using resistance bands, of which there are many different types. These can be used for general strength and conditioning and rehabilitation or injury prevention.

Resistance band exercises are ideal for home exercise programmes and can easily be incorporated into a circuit training format, helping to condition the cardiovascular system as well as strengthening specific muscle groups. Because resistance tubing is so compact and lightweight, it can easily be taken away on trips too.

FREE WEIGHTS

Using heavy weights on a regular basis may leave you stiff with slower dynamic movements, definitely not something you need if you're a surfer. It would be better to adopt a light weight, high rep workout, as this will build surfing strength and endurance – perfect for when it's six-foot and pumping and you need to get out back where the good stuff is!

If you are planning a resistance training programme then aim for basic progression. A well balanced training programme will cover all the major muscle groups; and always remember not to over train.

BASIC WEIGHT TRAINING

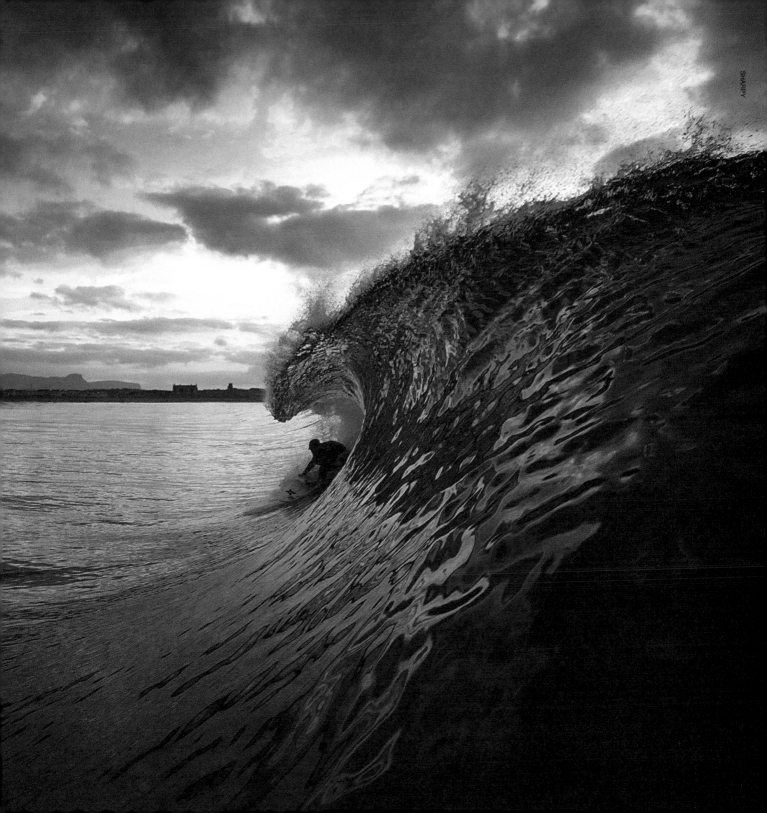

SHARPY

BASIC WEIGHT TRAINING EXERCISES

WITH ANY WEIGHTS PROGRAMME SOME KEY POINTS SHOULD BE TAKEN INTO CONSIDERATION:

Age If you are under 15 try to use own body weight exercises or resistance bands, and avoid lifting weights.

Plan out your session Look at an all over body programme, a well balanced programme is key to overall fitness and strength gains.

Keep a good tempo Tempo is the speed at which you lift the weight. In most gyms around the globe the majority of people lift at a pretty fast tempo, say a 1-2 seconds eccentric (negative or lowering) and a 1-2 seconds concentric (positive or raising).

Eat after your work out It is easy to forget to eat properly after training, try not to – a protein shake or cereal bar will keep you going until you have your next main meal.

Good training technique It's highly important not to rush your movements, this can cause injuries if you do.

Drink Don't forget that drinking during and after your workout is very important.

Rest Over training can take place if you do not take at least one day off a week.

Warm up Warm up and cool down for 5 to 10 minutes. Walking/jogging is a good way to warm up, then some mobility and stretching is an excellent way to cool down.

IT'S IMPORTANT TO STICK TO A STRUCTURED WORKOUT. REPS AND SETS ARE USED BY EXERCISE PROFESSIONALS AND ATHLETES AS THEY PROVIDE ORGANISATION AND STRUCTURE TO A WORKOUT. BY TRACKING YOUR SETS AND REPS YOU CAN SLOWLY INCREASE YOUR WORKOUT LOAD, THUS AVOIDING EXCESSIVE MUSCLE SORENESS.

TAKE A LOOK AT THE TRAINING PROGRAMMES TO SUIT YOUR LEVEL OF FITNESS WHICH STARTS ON PAGE 188

FRONT RAISES

Stand with feet about hip width apart, and a good upright posture.

Start with weights by your side, then, in line with your shoulders raise upwards to about shoulder high before repeating.

Aim for 6-8 reps

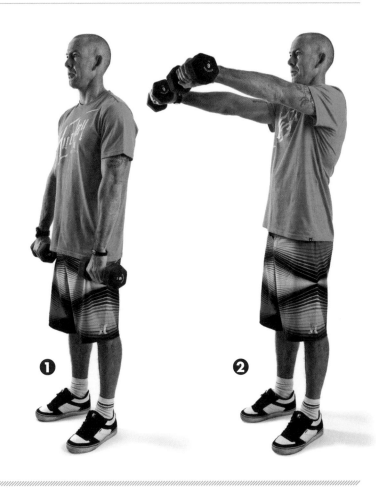

❶   **❷**

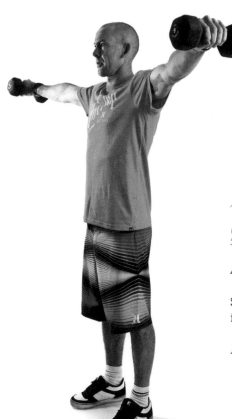

SIDE RAISE

Again stand with feet about hip width apart, and a good upright posture.

Start with weights by your side then, in line with your shoulders raise upwards in a lateral movement to about shoulder high before repeating.

Aim for 6-8 reps

SEATED SWISS BALL SHOULDER PRESS FROM BICEPS CURL

Aim for a good upright body position on the ball, feet about hip width apart.

Slowly, with elbows locked in against your body, perform a bicep curl.

From here push the weights upwards into a shoulder press. Keep your core tight during the movement. Lower and repeat.

8-10 reps then repeat

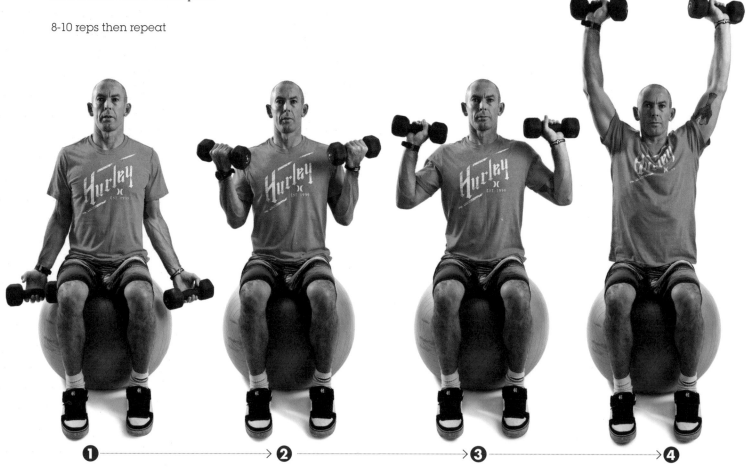

①   ②   ③   ④

BASIC SWISS BALL TRICEPS DROP

Start again on the ball, feet apart. Taking great care with the weight, squeeze the elbows together before lowering down behind your head.

With the weight lightly resting on the neck extend the weight upwards taking care NOT to lock the elbows to much.

8-10 reps then repeat

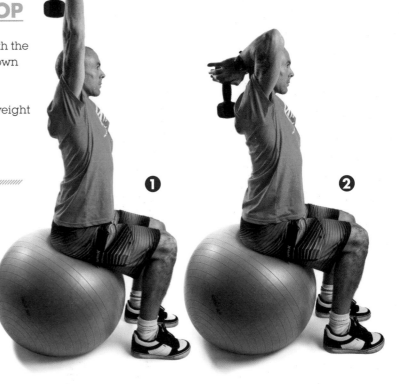

SQUATS WITH WEIGHTS

Try a few basic squats to start, shoulders back looking forwards, feet about hip width apart.

Then with weights in hands try a basic squat, push from heels and repeat.

6-10 reps

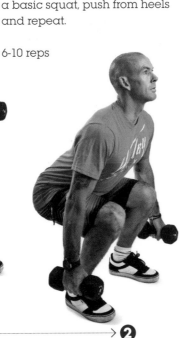

SWISS BALL SQUATS WITH WEIGHT

An alternative to the squat with weight is adding a Swiss Ball.

Stand tall sandwiching a Swiss Ball between you and a wall. Slowly squat, rolling the ball down the wall whilst keeping your back straight.

Push back up and repeat.

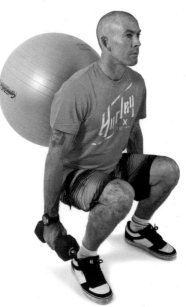

STANDING UPRIGHT ROWS

Start with feet a hips width apart with weights in hands.

Pull your elbows upwards, keep the weights close to your body, then repeat.

8-10 reps

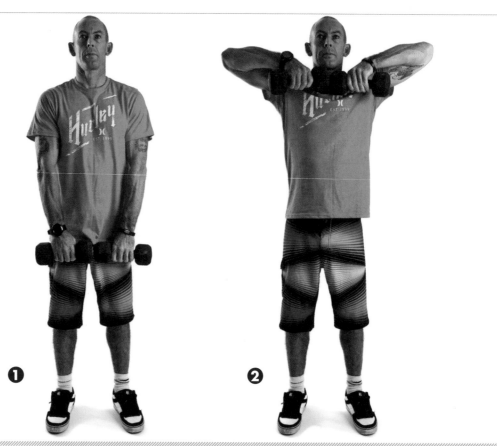

REVERSE FLY

Lean forwards with weights in hands, a hip width apart, soft knees.

Slowly raise weights in line with shoulders, squeezing the shoulder blades together.

4-6 reps

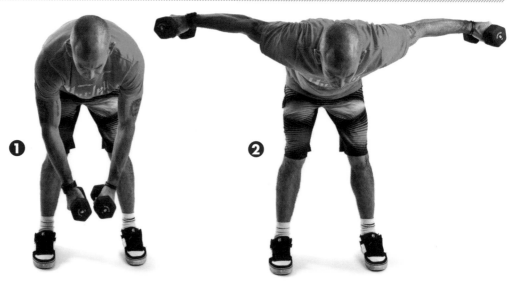

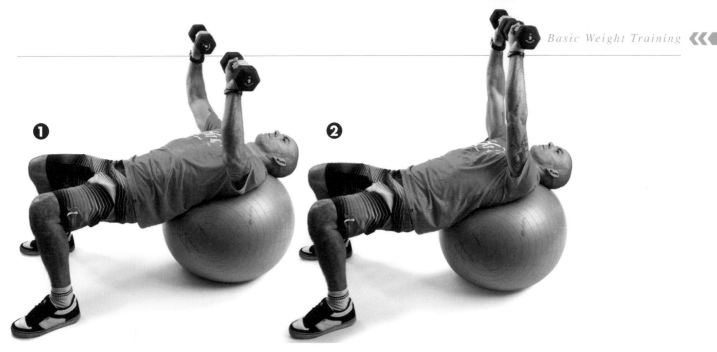

① **②**

SWISS BALL CHEST PRESS

Start by lying on the ball resting shoulders first, head supported.

From here bring the weights out to the sides, this will be backed up by the support from the ball.

Then keeping the core tight and hips up, raise the weights upwards to almost an extended arm. Repeat.

10-12 reps.

BASIC LUNGE WITH WEIGHTS

Start with both weights hanging down, shoulders back, look forward. Then step forward slowly, nice stride but not to far, both feet pointing forwards.

Aim for a ninety degree angle, shoulders back, then repeat on the other leg.

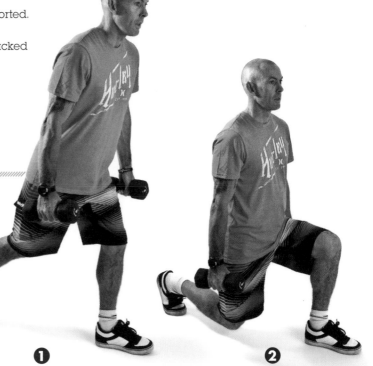

① **②**

BENEFITS OF TRIGGER POINT THERAPY

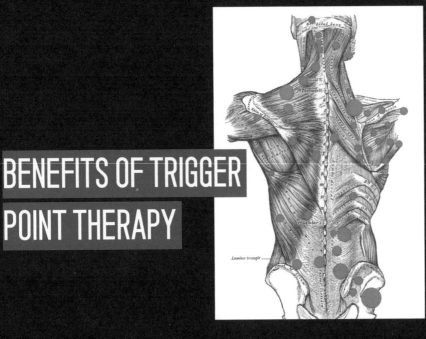

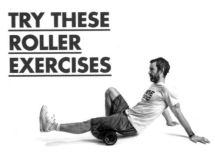

//HAMSTRING ROLL OUT
Place one leg on the roller with hips unsupported, then simply roll forwards slowly. Feet are crossed to increase leverage.

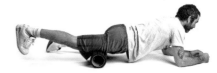

//QUADRICEPS ROLL OUT
Body is positioned prone with quadriceps on foam roller. It is very important to maintain proper core control as this will allow a safe body position.

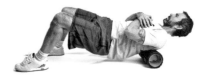

We all know that surfed out feeling. Adopt a regular Trigger Point myofascial release routine, and start to feel back to normal and relaxed in no time, ready for your next surf.

What is Trigger Point Therapy?
Based on the discoveries of Drs. Janet Travell and David Simons, myofascial Trigger Point Therapy is used to relieve muscular pain and dysfunction through applied pressure to trigger points of referred pain and through stretching exercises. These points are defined as localised areas in which the muscle and connective tissue are highly sensitive to pain when compressed. Pressure on these points can send referred pain to other specific parts of the body.

What are the benefits?
Trigger Point Therapy can relieve muscular aches and pains. It can also assist with the redevelopment of muscles and/or restore motion to joints.
• Improves joint range of motion
• Relieves muscle soreness and joint stress
• Corrects muscle imbalances
• Improves neuromuscular efficiency
• Maintains normal functional muscular length

//RHOMBOIDS AROUND THE SHOULDER BLADE
Surfers are prone to shoulder injuries and stiffness. The rhomboid muscles around the shoulder blades are often knotted. To start cross your arms to the opposite shoulder, to clear the shoulder blades across your thoracic wall. Then raise hips until they are unsupported. Make sure your head is in a neutral position. Roll back and forward.

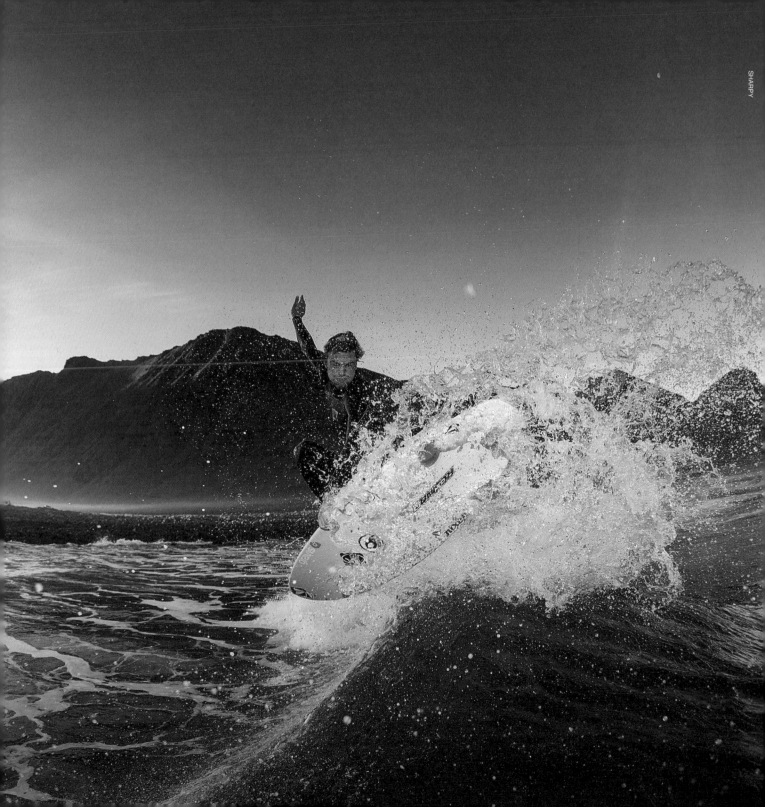

CORE STRENGTH TRAINING FOR SURFERS

What is core strength? The core muscles include your abdominals and back muscles plus those in your pelvic floor and hips. Many of your core muscles can't be seen because they're buried underneath other muscles. The transverse abdominals for example, are hiding underneath your rectus abdominals which hug the whole area below the belly button. While the rectus abdominals are sitting on top looking good, the transverse abdominals are working hard, especially during surfing movements.

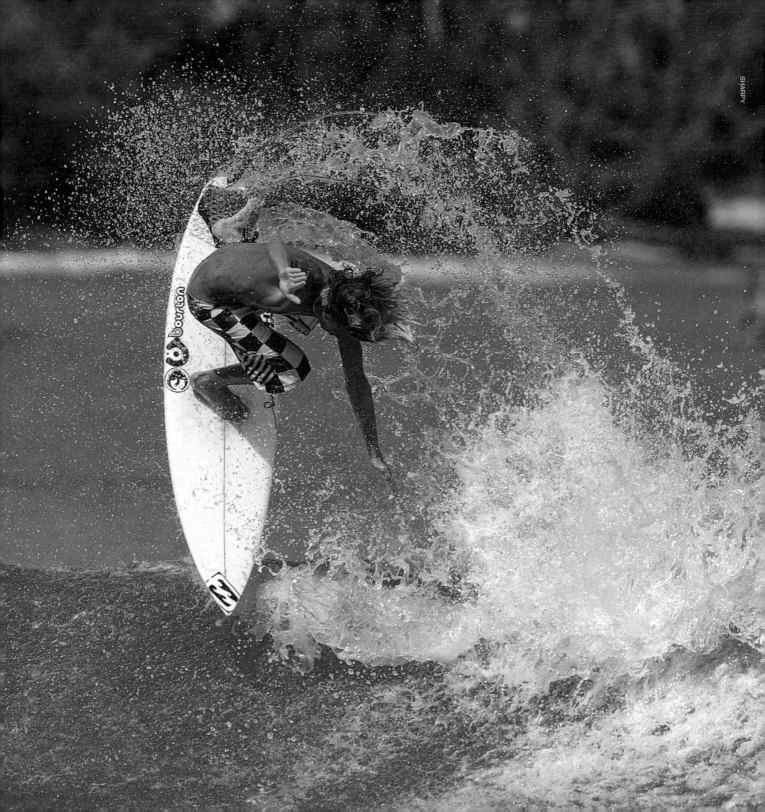

[THE TRANSVERSE ABDOMINALS
THE TRANSVERSE ABDOMINALS ARE A KEY FACTOR IN CORE STRENGTH AND A STRONG CORE IS VITAL DURING SURFING MOVEMENTS]

CORE STRENGTH TRAINING AND ATHLETIC PERFORMANCE

The muscles of the trunk and torso stabilise the spine from the pelvis to the neck and shoulder – they allow the transfer of powerful movements of the arms and legs.

Training the muscles of the core also serves to correct postural imbalances which can lead to injuries. The biggest benefit of core training is to develop functional fitness – that is fitness which is essential to both daily living and regular activities.

Core strengthening exercises are most effective when the torso works as a solid unit and both front and back muscles contract at the same time, multi joint movements are performed, and stabilisation of the spine is monitored.

DECADE3D/SHUTTERSTOCK.COM

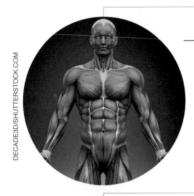

RECTUS ABDOMINALS

Located along the front of the abdomen, this is the most well known abdominal muscle and is often referred to as the "six pack" due to its appearance in fit and thin individuals.

The rectus abdominals help to flex the spinal column, narrowing the space between the pelvis and the ribs. They are also active during side bending motions, and also help to stabilise the trunk during surfing movements.

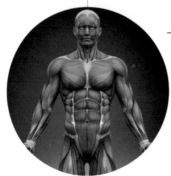

EXTERNAL OBLIQUE MUSCLES

The next group of muscles that make up the abdominals are the external oblique muscles. This pair of muscles is located on each side of the rectus abdominals. The muscle fibres of the external obliques run diagonally downward and inward from the lower ribs to the pelvis, forming a V shape.

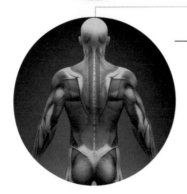

ERECTOR SPINE

This group of three muscles runs along your neck to your lower back. The erector spine muscles support your spinal column and promote ease of mobility, encourage correct posture during surfing paddling movements, and aid support.

This large muscular mass varies in size and structure at different parts of the vertebra column.

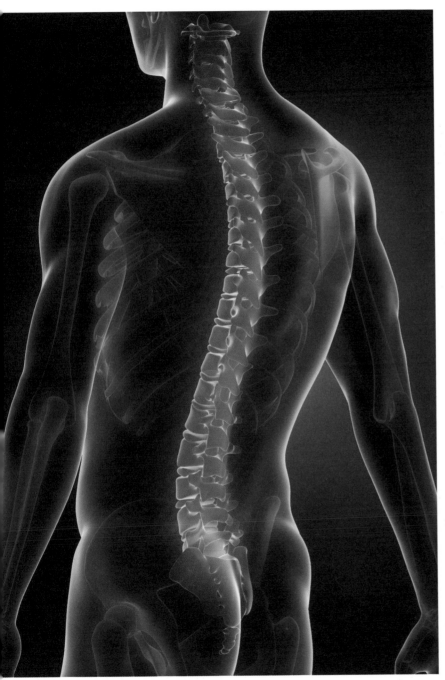

YOUR NEUTRAL SPINE ALIGNMENT

Standing in front of a mirror you will notice your lower back is not flat, but has a slight curve. When your back is in neutral spine alignment the ligaments, muscles and discs are at their optimal position and under the least stress.

Feet should be shoulder width apart. Thigh muscles elongated without locking the knees back.

Maintain a small hollow in your lower back. Avoid the tendency for too much arch/leaning back, especially with prolonged standing. The "tail" should remain slightly tucked down.

Lift the breastbone. As you do this, the shoulder blades will move down the back. This should create a good distance from your hipbone to your rib cage.

Make your chin level. The highest point of your body should be the top back region of your head. Relax your jaw and neck muscles.

SUMMARY

- Always maintain a good posture.
- Core training can be done every day.
- If you suffer from back problems some core exercises might not be suitable always consult a doctor if you're unsure.
- Always work within your capabilities.

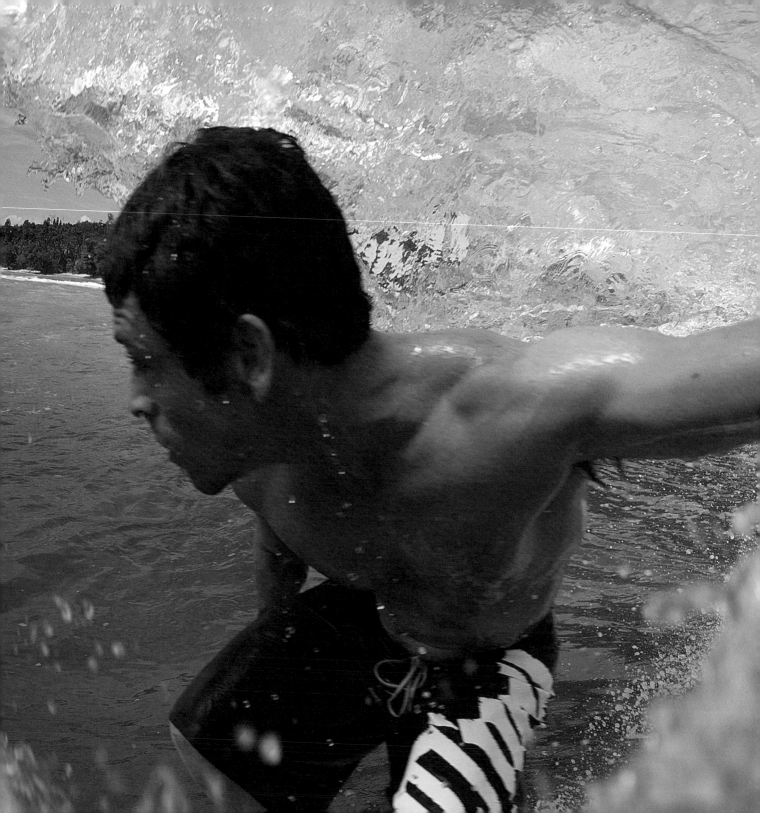

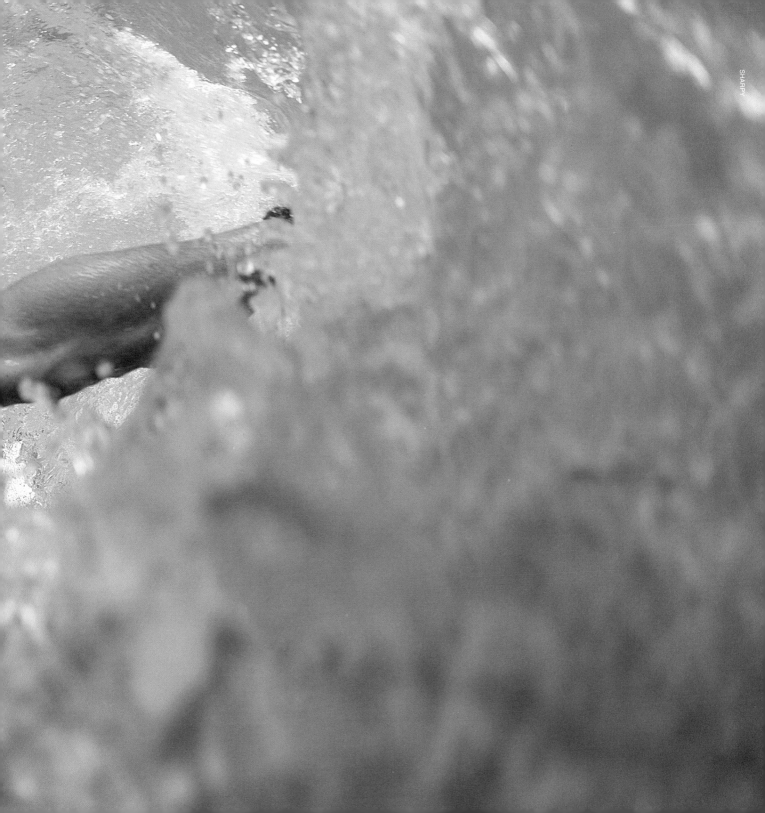

CORE EXERCISES

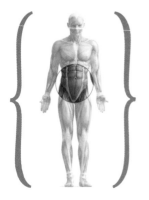

As you begin to lower into a compressed body position at the bottom of the wave there are certain specific demands on your body. For example, your core engages as you begin to lean into the wave. As you hold your compressed body position your leg strength is then put to the test with the knees, ankles and even the soles of your feet coming in to play.

SWISS BALL PLANK - BEGINNERS

Start this exercise with elbows on the Swiss ball, keep your head in line with your spine, legs slightly apart and use your arms to support your body. Hold the position.

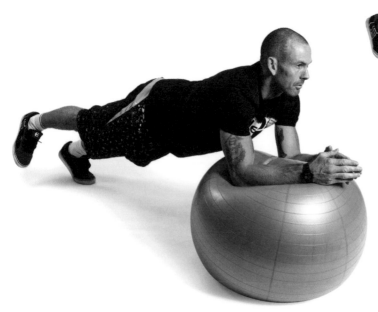

SWISS BALL PLANK WITH LEG LIFT - INTERMEDIATE

Start this exercise in the same way as the basic plank, only this time try lifting one foot off the ground, just for a few seconds, to overload your core and then swap to the other side.

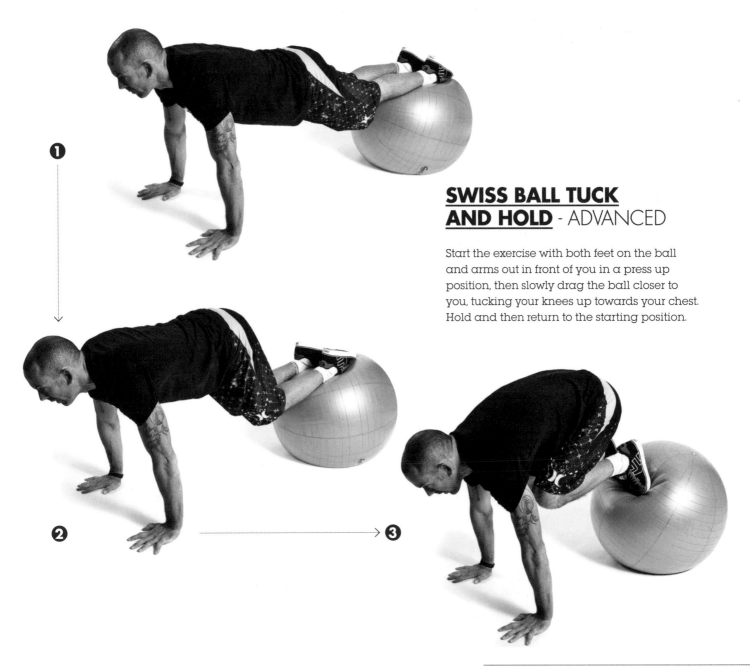

SWISS BALL TUCK AND HOLD - ADVANCED

Start the exercise with both feet on the ball and arms out in front of you in a press up position, then slowly drag the ball closer to you, tucking your knees up towards your chest. Hold and then return to the starting position.

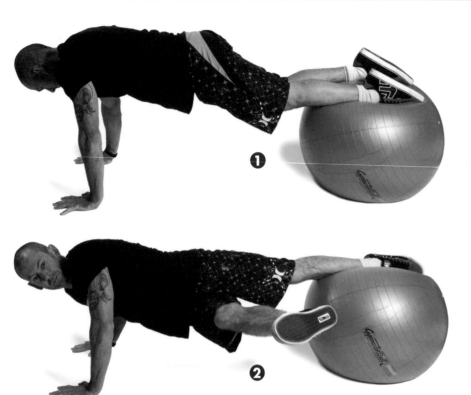

SWISS BALL LEG KICK OUT - ADVANCED

This is a great exercise for upper body strength and the core!

Start the exercise in a press up position, feet on the ball, then remove one leg and cross it over to the other side of the body.

Hold and then place back on the ball before repeating.

BASIC CRUNCH - BEGINNERS

This will strengthen your abdominals. Start by placing your hands on your thighs, then simply run your hands upwards towards your knees.

Then lower slowly back down again before repeating.

Try 10 reps.

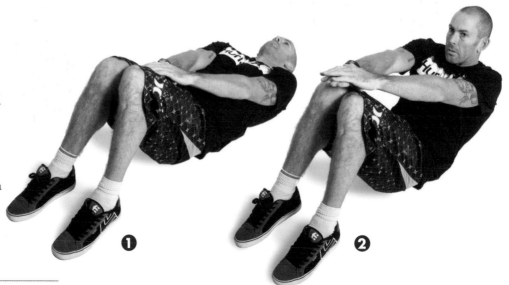

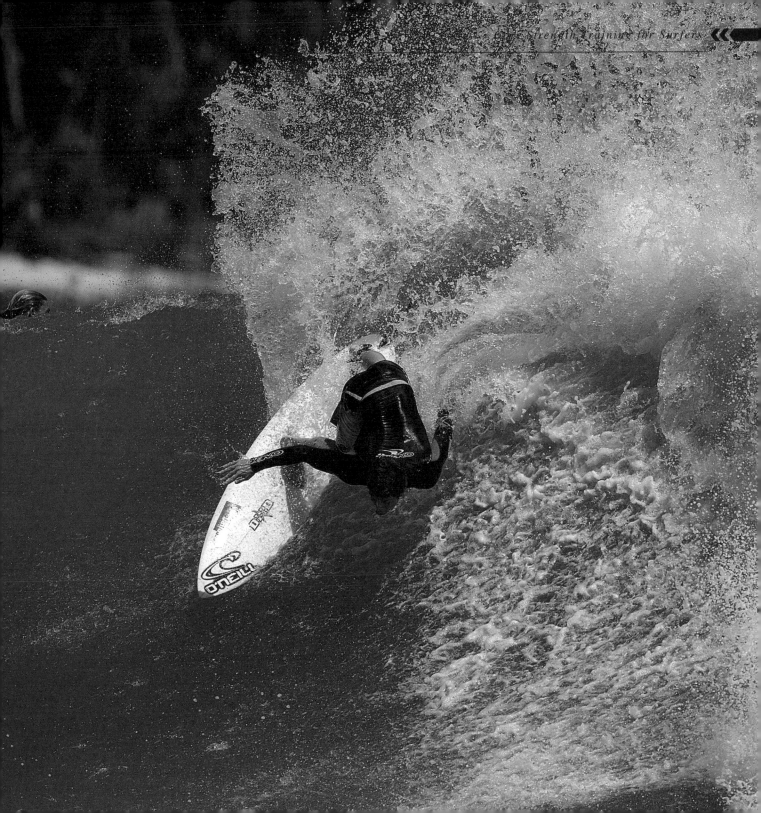

PADDLE POWER

There are many aspects to boosting your surfing paddle power. General aerobic fitness is important, as are upper body strength exercises. The primary muscles groups used are the muscles around the shoulder blades, posterior and anterior. Shoulder muscles, a strong core and strong lower back muscles help to stabilise the movements.

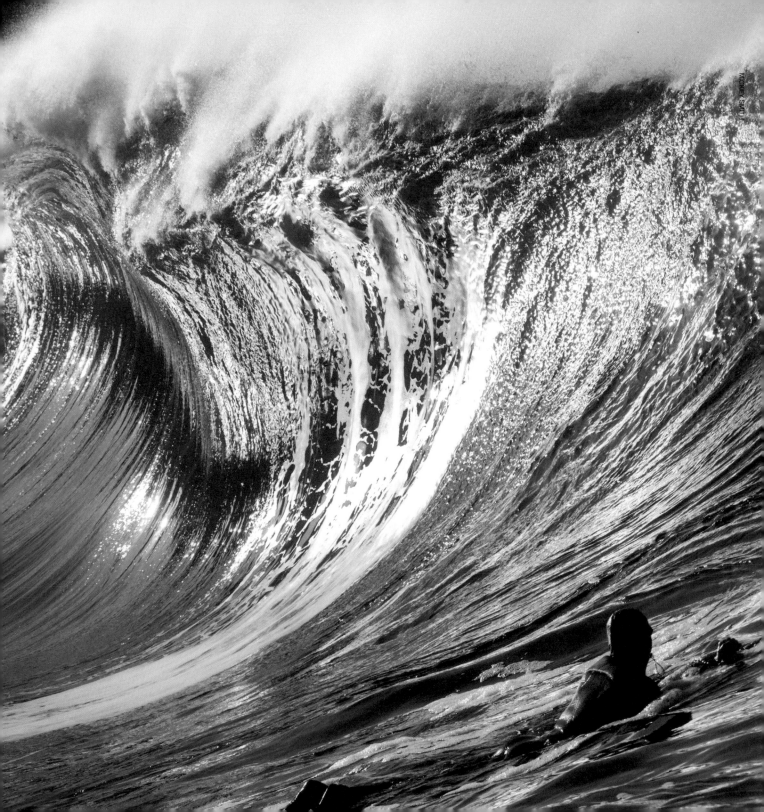

PADDLE POWER TRAINING

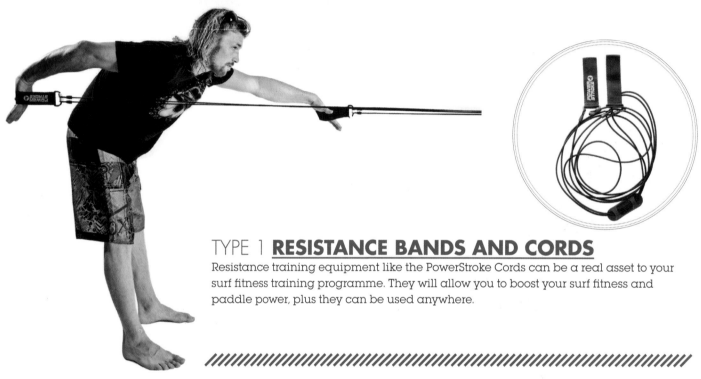

TYPE 1 **RESISTANCE BANDS AND CORDS**

Resistance training equipment like the PowerStroke Cords can be a real asset to your surf fitness training programme. They will allow you to boost your surf fitness and paddle power, plus they can be used anywhere.

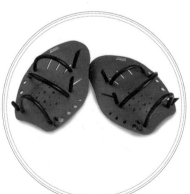

TYPE 2 **SWIMMING TRAINING AIDS**

In the world of swimming, many swimmers – from recreational to elite – use swim hand paddles. These can be a real asset to the surfer looking for improvements in surfing paddle power. Hand paddles boost the muscles used in surfing paddle outs and wave catching. There are many different types and sizes (for more information go to Fit4swimming.com).

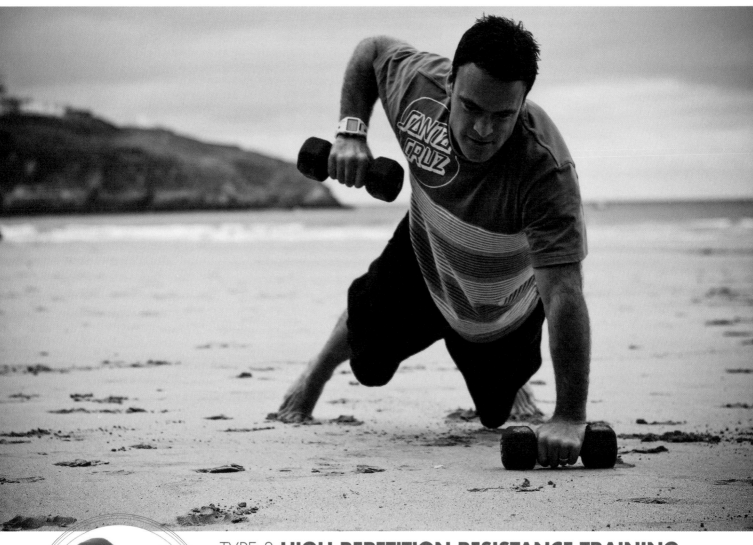

TYPE 3 **HIGH REPETITION RESISTANCE TRAINING**

Using free weights to improve strength and endurance is also a great way to increase your paddle power. Isolating the muscle groups that are used during the paddle out or wave catching will see improvements, and used in conjunction with resistance cords will see significant gains.

THE POWERSTROKE CORD

Boosting your paddle power is a must. The PowerStroke cord can be used here to isolate the muscle groups used for paddling into that perfect wave. One of the most important muscle groups involved with paddling is the back of the arms – the muscle group known as the triceps.

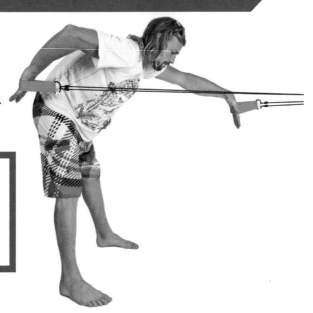

> FOR SPRINT TRAINING TRY 10X20 SECONDS FAST WITH 30 SECONDS REST AFTER EACH 20 SECOND SPRINT

Example PowerStroke Cord Workouts:

BEGINNER

Do 5x60 seconds at a moderate pace with light breathing. Paddle slowly with smooth controlled movements. After each 60 seconds of paddle take 30 seconds rest.

After 2 minutes of rest try 4x2 minutes of paddle taking 30 seconds rest.

And finally try 3x3 minutes of paddle taking 45 seconds rest after each 3 minutes.

Cool down with 10 minutes light stretching.

INTERMEDIATE

Warm up 5 minutes mobility exercises.

5x2 minutes light paddle with 30 seconds rest after each 2 minutes. Then do 4x3 minutes with 30 seconds rest after each 30 seconds.

And finally try 1x5 minutes non-stop light paddle.

Cool down with 10 minutes light stretching.

ADVANCED

Warm up with 5 minutes mobility exercises.

10x2 minutes light paddle with 30 seconds rest after each 2 minutes.

Then do 5x4 minutes at a strong to moderate pace with 60 seconds rest after each 4 minutes.

Also try a 10 minute non-stop paddle.

Cool down with 10 minutes light stretching.

POWERSTROKE CORD TRICEPS EXTENSION

Start the exercise by attaching your PowerStroke Cord around something secure. The cord should be about head high and in line with your shoulders.

Kneel on the floor with your hands in the handles, then take the handles above your head, elbows close together. Slowly start the movement from the back of the neck and extend your arms upwards as you do so, working the back of the arms.

Make sure the PowerStroke Cord generates resistance, but not too far away that movement becomes impossible. Try 10 reps then rest before attempting another 10.

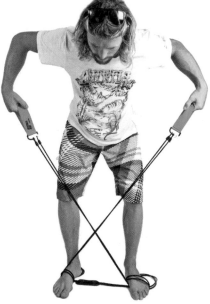

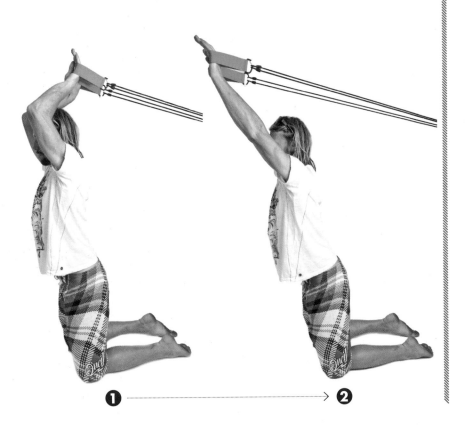

❶ ⟶ ❷

POWERSTROKE REVERSE FLY

Standing with feet firmly on the cords, grab both handles, then with a relaxed neck, slowly draw the arms outwards.

From here squeeze the shoulder blades together, repeat 8-10 times .

Rest before attempting another 10.

EXPLOSIVE POWER

Explosive leg power in surfing is a highly desirable commodity, whether you're charging off the lip or simply popping up onto your board, especially in less powerful summer waves. Plyometric training may be just what you need to get you into bombs that little bit earlier, or to boost your summer wave count.

Plyometrics is a type of exercise training designed to produce fast, powerful movements, and this in turn will improve the functions of the nervous system, generally for the purpose of improving performance in sports. Plyometric movements in which a muscle is loaded and then contracted in rapid sequence, use the strength, elasticity and innervations of muscle and surrounding tissues to jump higher, run faster, throw further, or hit harder, depending on the training goal.

There can be different intensities with plyometric training, from basic skipping to vertical jumps, bounding, single leg jumps or box jumps. In addition to gaining explosive power, plyometric training will improve the ligaments, tendons and muscles of the legs, which can help in injury prevention.

Before any plyometric training session it is highly advisable to follow a basic warm up of at least 10 minutes. You should aim to build your sessions up to at least 20 minutes, two to three times a week, for the best results.

Plyometrics (and any impact exercise) can increase the risk of injury if you don't follow certain safety precautions. The tremendous force generated during these moves requires that athletes use them sparingly and with proper training.

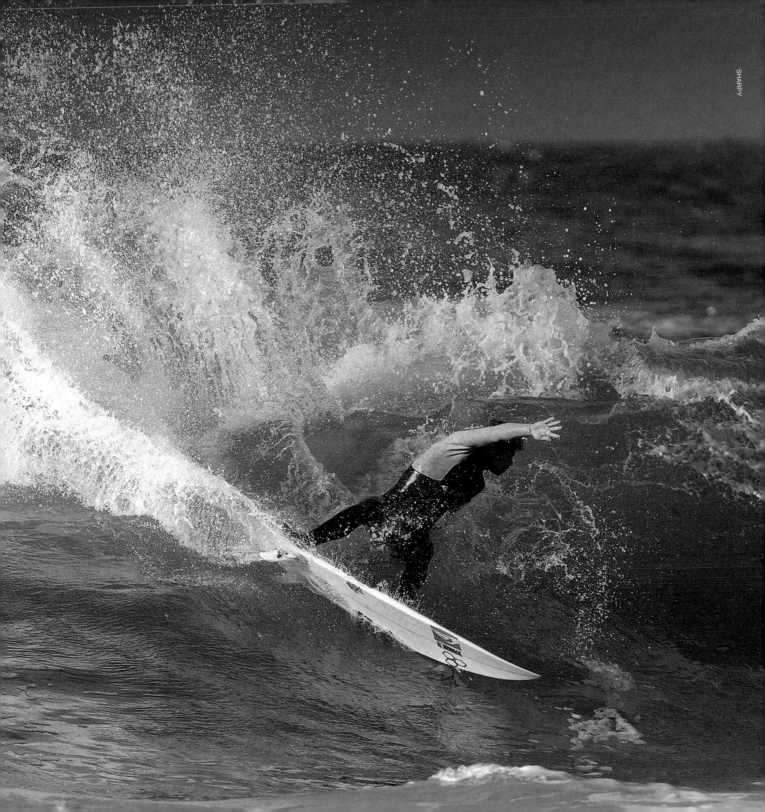

VERTICAL JUMP
EXERCISES

Start the exercise by standing with your feet a hip width apart. Remember, using a soft surface is very important. Once you are happy with your stance, do just one powerful jump upwards, try to take 5 seconds rest between each jump. Try 5 jumps then rest before repeating another set.

SINGLE LEG VERTICAL JUMPS - BEGINNERS

Start the move with legs at 90 degree angle then, with one big powerful movement, bring your knee up to your chest using your arms to aid the movement and add balance.

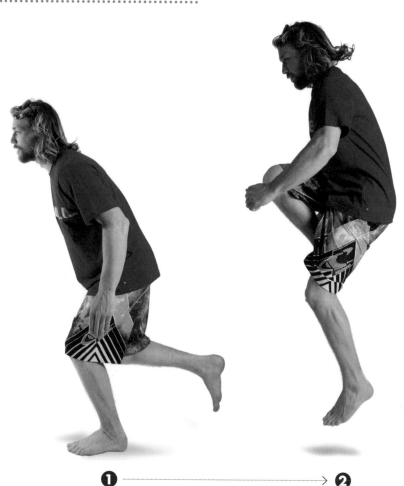

❶ - > **❷**

SINGLE LEG JUMPS WITH LIGHT WEIGHT
- INTERMEDIATE

Start the move in the same way as before only this time holding light weights which will add resistance throughout the move.

SINGLE LEG JUMPS WITH HEAVY WEIGHT
- ADVANCED

Complete the move as before only using a heavy weight. (This is not advised if you are new to exercise or you have not yet developed to an intermediate level of strength to try this exercise.)

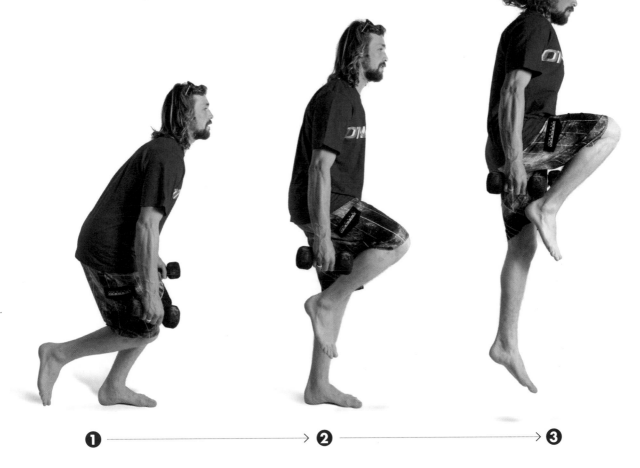

❶ ⟶ ❷ ⟶ ❸

GAIN MORE EXPLOSIVE POWER FROM USING AN EXERCISE STEP

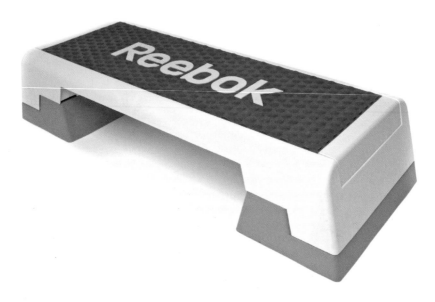

THE EXERCISE STEP, ALTHOUGH A VERY BASIC BIT OF TRAINING KIT, IS HIGHLY VERSATILE. IT CAN BE USED FOR A WHOLE RANGE OF EXERCISES FOR SURF FITNESS TRAINING, FROM THE VERY SIMPLE TO THE ADVANCED, AEROBIC AND ANAEROBIC TRAINING, STRENGTH TRAINING, AND EVEN CORE AND BALANCE TRAINING.

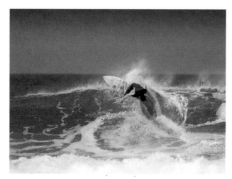
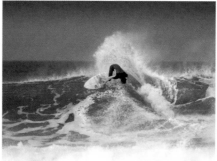
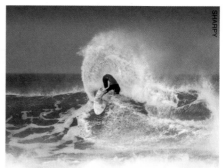

SHARPY

BASIC STEP UP

The basic step is simply a step up, but can be used at pace to improve aerobic fitness, and leg strength.

Start by stepping one foot first on the step then the other on top of the platform then stepping the first foot back on the floor with the second following.

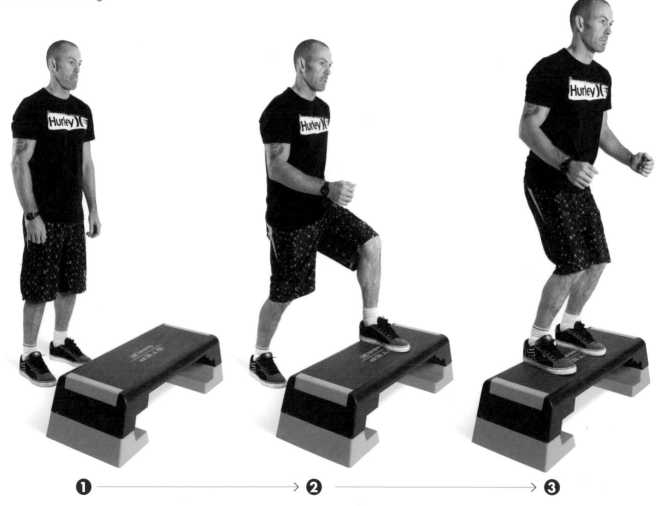

❶   ❷   ❸

SIDE STEPS AT PACE

The Reebok side step is also a basic exercise but can be used to boost aerobic and anaerobic fitness and improve coordination when done at speed.

Simply start the exercise with feet both sides of the step then, slowly to start, step one foot up on the box followed by the other. As your coordination improves increase speed. As you progress with your fitness and the exercise speeds up, intensify your step over with a jump.

Work at intervals, improving your fitness by increasing your duration. (20, 30, 40 seconds etc.)

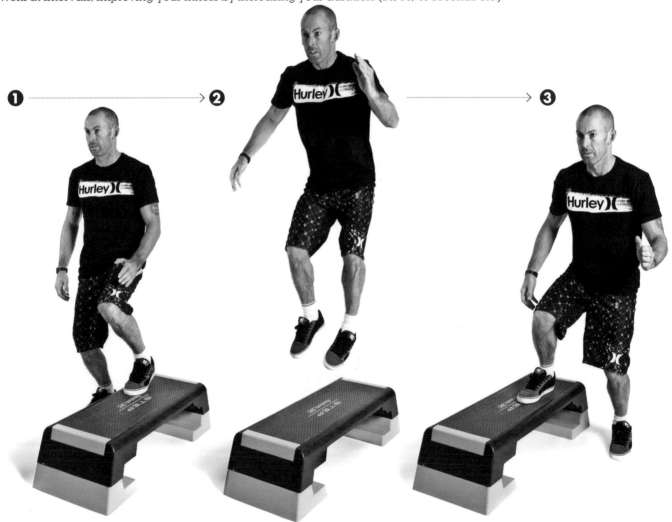

SUPER LUNGES WITH WEIGHTS

Leg strength in surfing movements is very important and sharper movements can be gained from an improvement in leg strength.

Step forward with weights hanging downwards, then from there raise legs upwards, back down to start position.

Repeat 8 times.

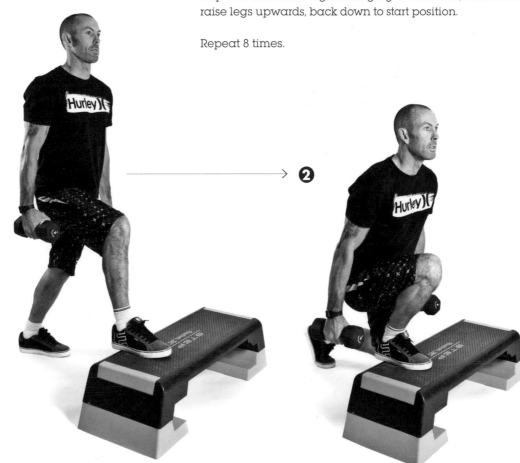

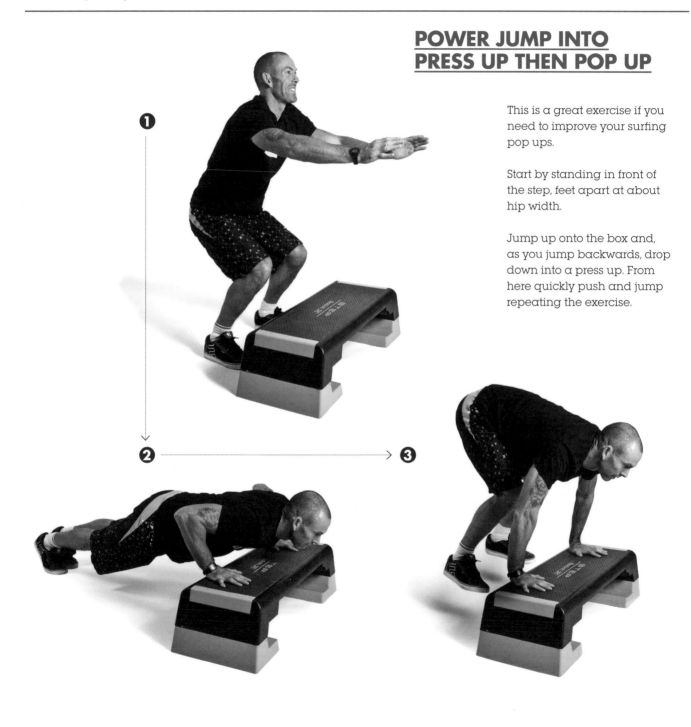

POWER JUMP INTO PRESS UP THEN POP UP

This is a great exercise if you need to improve your surfing pop ups.

Start by standing in front of the step, feet apart at about hip width.

Jump up onto the box and, as you jump backwards, drop down into a press up. From here quickly push and jump repeating the exercise.

BOX JUMP - BEGINNERS

For this exercise you will need a box or similar step that's about knee high. It's important to stay well focused during the movement to avoid injury.

Start with both feet slightly apart then, using your arms, jump up and onto the box and back down onto the floor again before repeating.

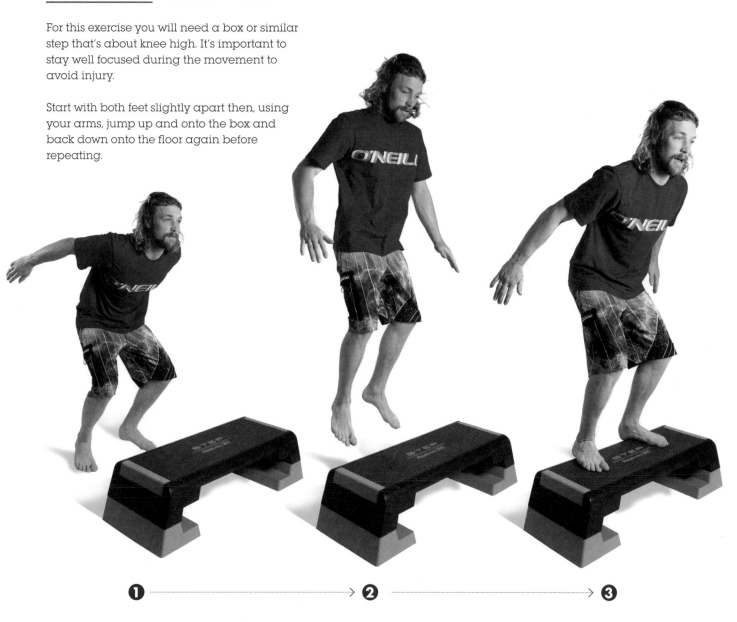

① ----------> **②** ----------> **③**

BOX JUMP WITH MEDICINE BALL - INTERMEDIATE

This is definitely much harder than a basic box jump so take care during the move and start with a very light ball.

Stand with both feet about a hip width apart and with both hands on the ball, then jump onto the box throwing the ball upwards as you do, but keeping hold of it at the same time.

As you reach the top of the box you should have your ball over your head.

BOX JUMP WITH MEDICINE BALL (HEAVY) - ADVANCED

For this exercise simply use a much heavier ball but take additional care as the extra weight will generate instability during the move.

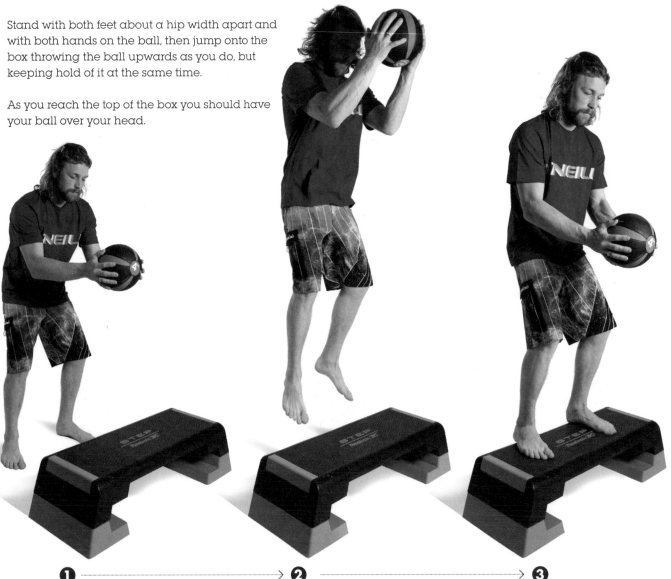

❶ ⟶ **❷** ⟶ **❸**

JUMP AND STICK - ADVANCED

Grab a Bosu and try a jump and stick exercise. This can improve your coordination and explosive power. Make certain the Bosu is securely fixed and will not move, then use all your power to jump upwards and stick on top of the Bosu.

Once you land hold a squat position and and then repeat 10 times.

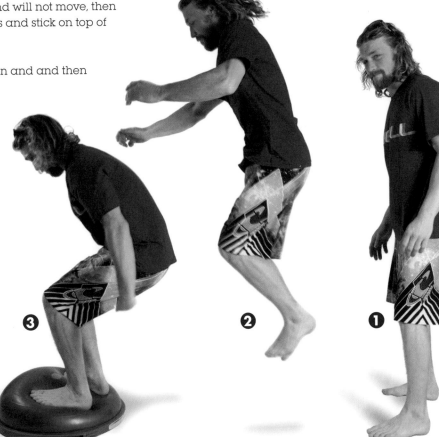

❸ ❷ ❶

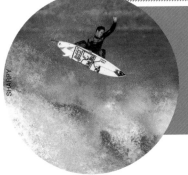

SHARPY

PLYOMETRICS FOR EXPLOSIVE SURFING POWER

BY USING HIGH-QUALITY AND MULTI-DIRECTIONAL DRILLS, EXPLOSIVE MOVEMENT AND RESPONSE TIMES CAN BE IMPROVED. SPEED AND AGILITY ARE UNDOUBTABLY HIGHLY DESIRABLE QUALITIES IN ALL SURFING MOVEMENTS. BASIC PLYOMETRIC TRAINING IN YOUR TRAINING PROGRAMME WILL SHARPEN YOUR SURFING MOVEMENTS MAKING THEM FASTER.

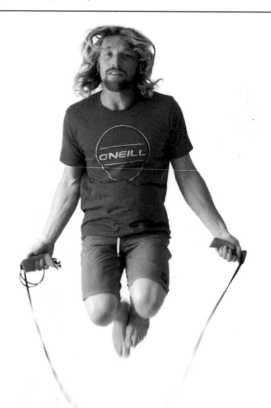

SKIPPING - BEGINNERS TO ADVANCED

Skipping can be really great for a surfer's fitness. Done on a regular basis for at least 20-30 minutes it will really help build strength in the legs, and improve the cardio vascular fitness.

Try these simple sets

• Warm up: 5-8 minutes

• 12x30 seconds steady skip with 20 seconds rest.

• 8x60 seconds strong skipping with 60 seconds rest.

• 12x20 seconds super fast with 20 seconds rest.

Many competitive swimmers use skipping as a great way to warm up before hitting the water for the pool based warm up.

SKIPPING CAN REALLY HELP A SURFER GET READY FOR A HEAT. YOU MAY NOT THINK SO OR EVEN WISH TO LET YOUR FELLOW COMPETITORS SEE YOU SKIPPING BEFORE YOU HIT YOUR HEAT, BUT YOU WILL BE SIGNIFICANTLY MORE READY TO SURF. JUST STICK TO LIGHT SKIPPING, 3-5 MINS WORTH.

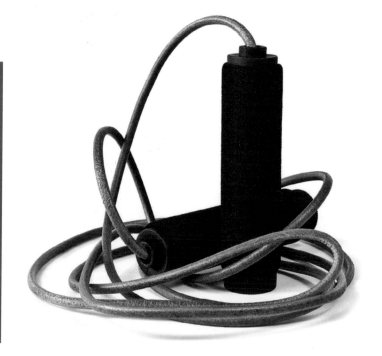

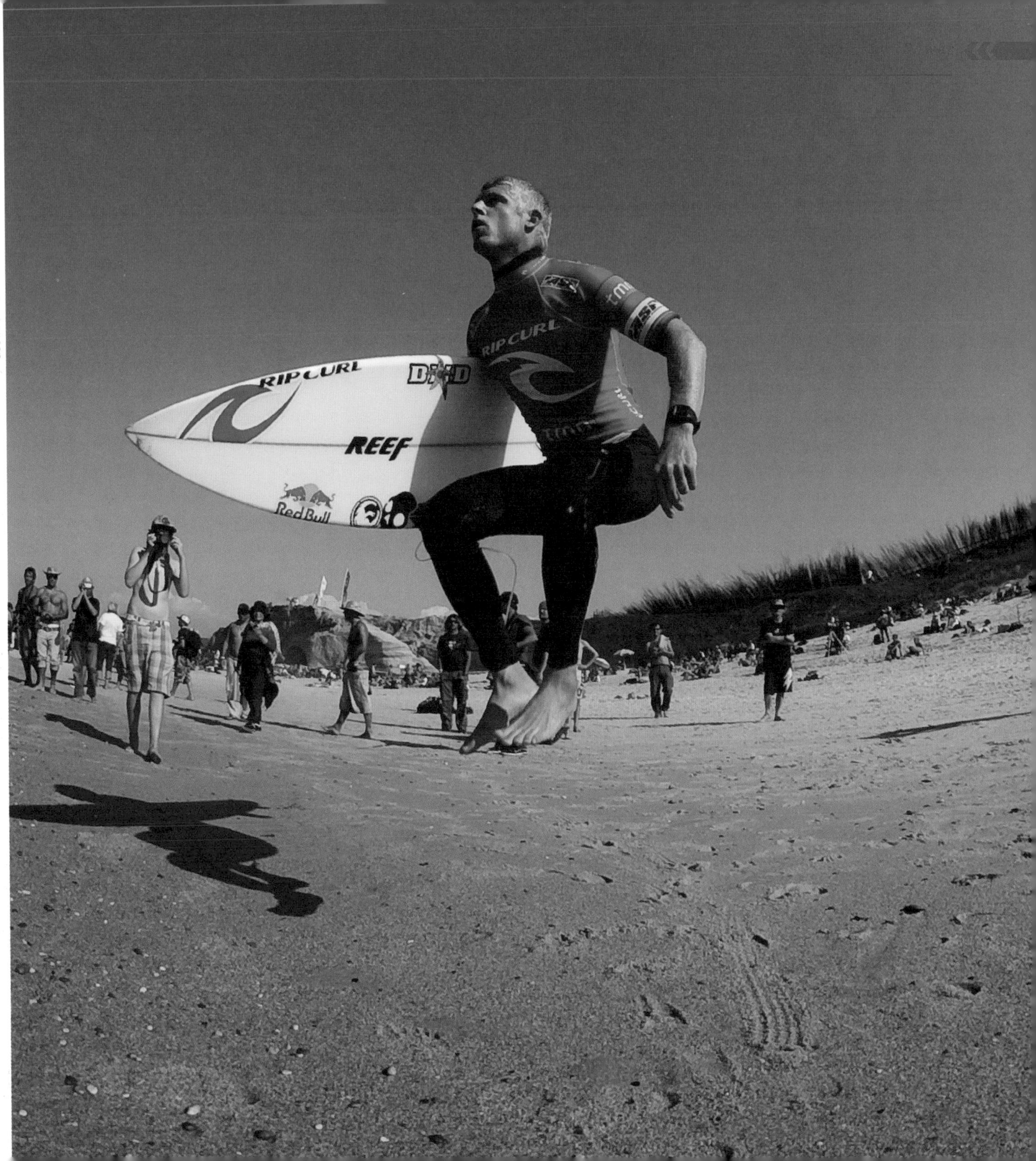

GUSTAVO MIGUEL FERNANDES / SHUTTERSTOCK.COM

FOREHAND AND BACKHAND BOTTOM TURN

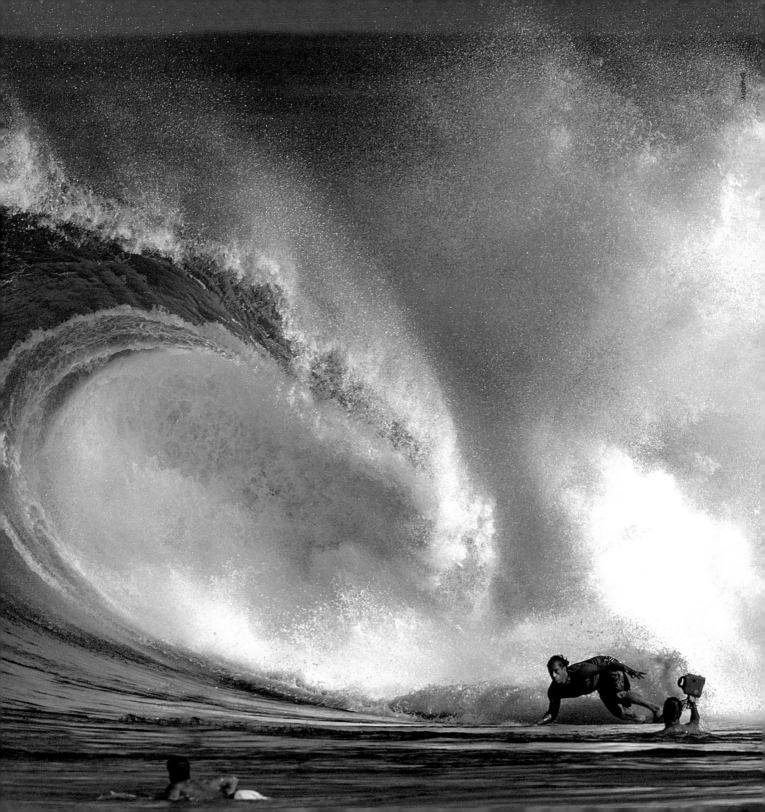

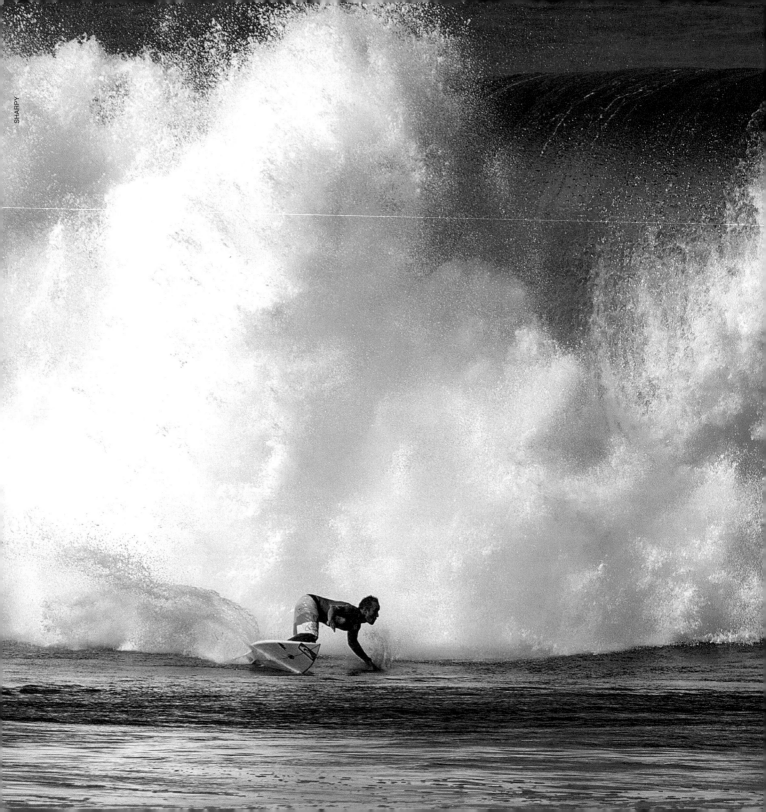

SHARPY

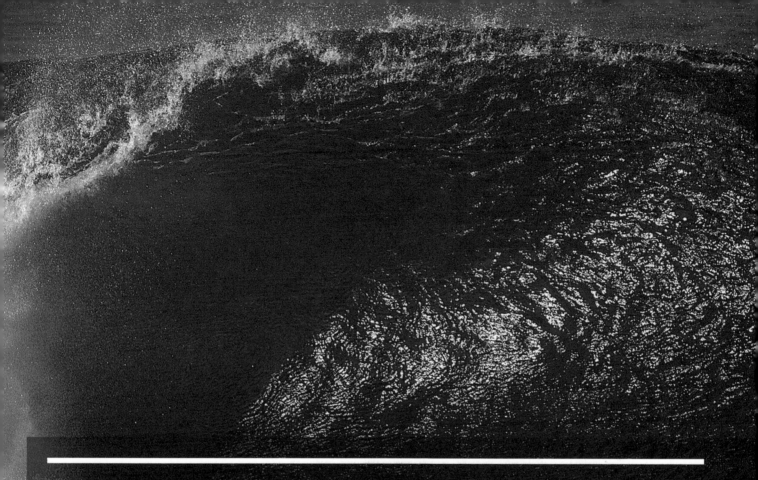

The bottom turn is probably the most important manoeuvre in surfing, a manoeuvre that generates speed and drive while setting the surfer up for his next move on the wave. It allows the surfer to get around long sections or vertically hit the lip.

As you drive up the lip of the wave your glutes (buttocks) aid in the movement, then as you begin to lean back into the next movement your legs work alongside your core, which allows you to stay in contact with the board. Many surf training exercises will involve a lot of balance, and proprioception (the body's ability to realise its place in space, in this case on a surfboard) plays a major role in training for improvements in progressive performance surfing.

If a surfer is moving into a position that could sprain their ankle, improved proprioception will decrease the risk by alerting the athlete to the danger.

Improvements in proprioception can also improve a surfer's overall performance by improving balance and awareness, and enabling the surfer to control their body movements more effectively.

During a surfing movement like a forehand bottom turn, there is a lot of down force onto the board to bring about the movement. The muscles that are involved, if strengthened, will then bring about more power. For a sharper movement it is important to target those muscles.

OBLIQUES EXERCISES

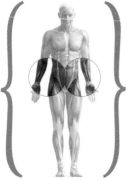

As you begin to lower into a compressed body position at the bottom of the wave, there are specific demands on your body. For example, your core engages as you begin to lean into the wave. As you hold your compressed body position your leg strength is then put to the test with the knees, ankles and even the soles of your feet coming in to play.

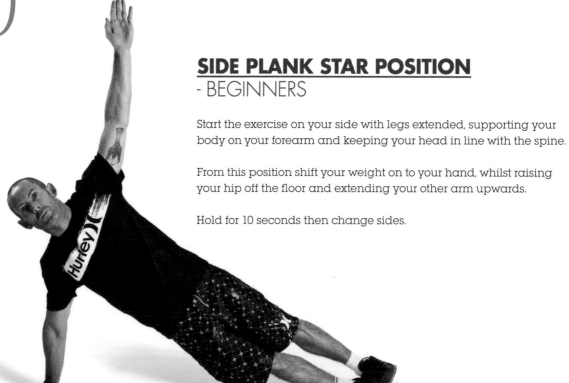

SIDE PLANK STAR POSITION
- BEGINNERS

Start the exercise on your side with legs extended, supporting your body on your forearm and keeping your head in line with the spine.

From this position shift your weight on to your hand, whilst raising your hip off the floor and extending your other arm upwards.

Hold for 10 seconds then change sides.

SIDE PLANK STAR POSITION WITH LEG RAISE - INTERMEDIATE

This is basically the same exercise as the beginner's star, only this time once you are in the correct position lift one leg upward, about 3 inches off from the other one, and hold.

SIDE PLANK STAR POSITION USING BOSU - ADVANCED

For the advanced exercise you will need a Bosu Balance Trainer or an Indo Board with Gigante cushion – start the exercise in the same way as before only this time place one hand on the centre of the Bosu Balance Trainer.

The added challenge will come with the instability of the Bosu or Indo Board.

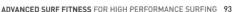

LOWER ABDOMINAL
EXERCISES

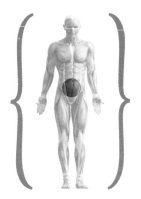

LEG RISES - BEGINNERS

Lie on your back with your hands alongside your hips, put your legs together and slowly raise your feet 6 inches off the floor. As you do so pull your belly button inwards, this will help keep your lower back from arching.

Hold for as long as you can, keeping your back to the floor. 4-6 reps.

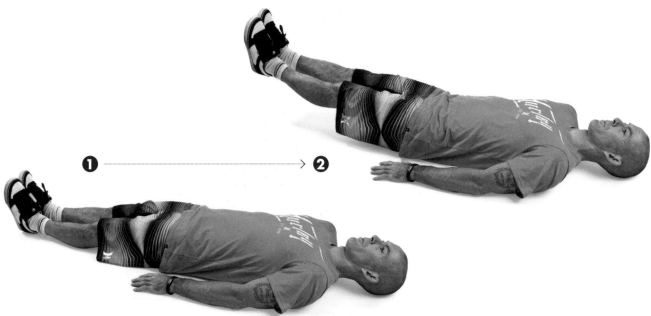

❶ ....➤ ❷

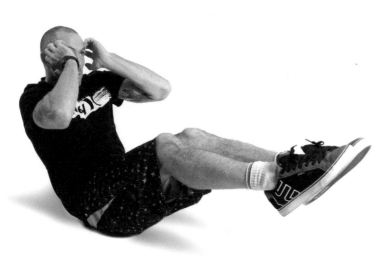

REVERSE CRUNCHES WITH SIDE BEND - INTERMEDIATE

Lie on the floor with your arms placed by your side, then slowly bring the knees in towards the chest until they're bent to 90 degrees, with feet together or crossed.

Contract your abs to curl the hips off the floor, reaching your legs up towards the ceiling. After each upwards movement add a side to side movement.

Note: You can advance the move by adding ankle weights to increase resistance.

CRUNCHES WITH MEDICINE BALL - ADVANCED

Start the exercise with a basic crunch only this time use a medicine ball to increase the resistance. Hold the ball on your chest through the move. As you get stronger try adding a twist to the routine. After each forwards movement take the ball round to each hip in the form of a twist.

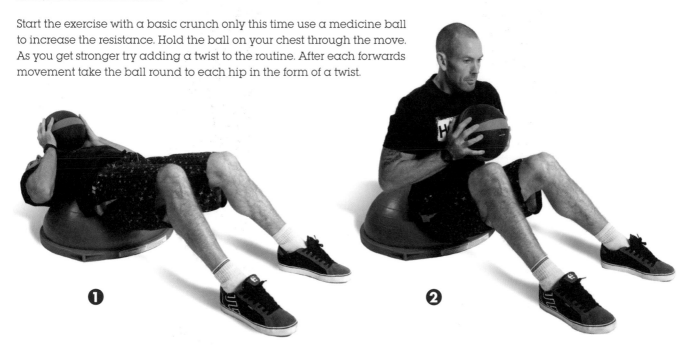

❶ ❷

KNEE & ANKLE
EXERCISES

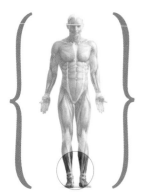

At some point many surfers will have injured a knee or ankle. Strong ankles and knees are vital for improved performance and injury prevention.

BALL THROWS BALANCE AND CATCH
- INTERMEDIATE

Start the exercise by standing on one leg on an Indo board and Gigante cushion. Get a partner to throw you a ball, the ball should be thrown left, right and high up – for the best results try 20 reps and then repeat on the other side.

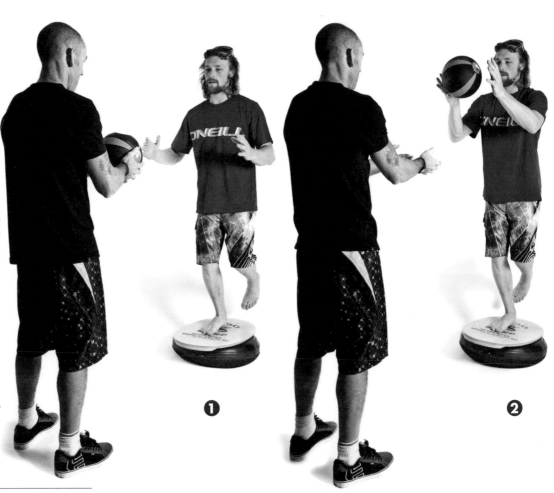

❶ ❷

INDO BOARD AND GIGANTE SINGLE LEG SQUATS - ADVANCED

If you don't have an Indo Board you can try this with the flat side of a BOSU Balance Trainer. This exercise can also be done just on its own if you're finding the Indo squat too tricky at first.

Position yourself in the centre of the deck, maintain a good posture and a slightly bent leg. Once you have found a good balance try slowly squatting down, then try a one second pause before coming back up. Aim for a 90 degree angle in your leg.

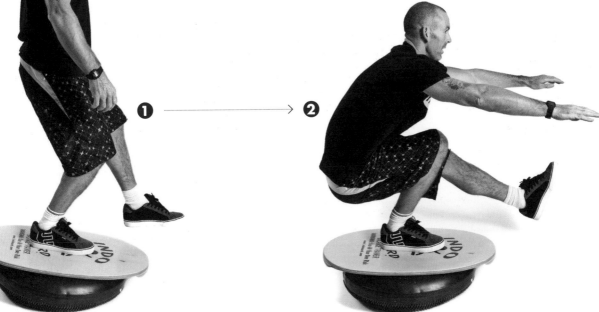

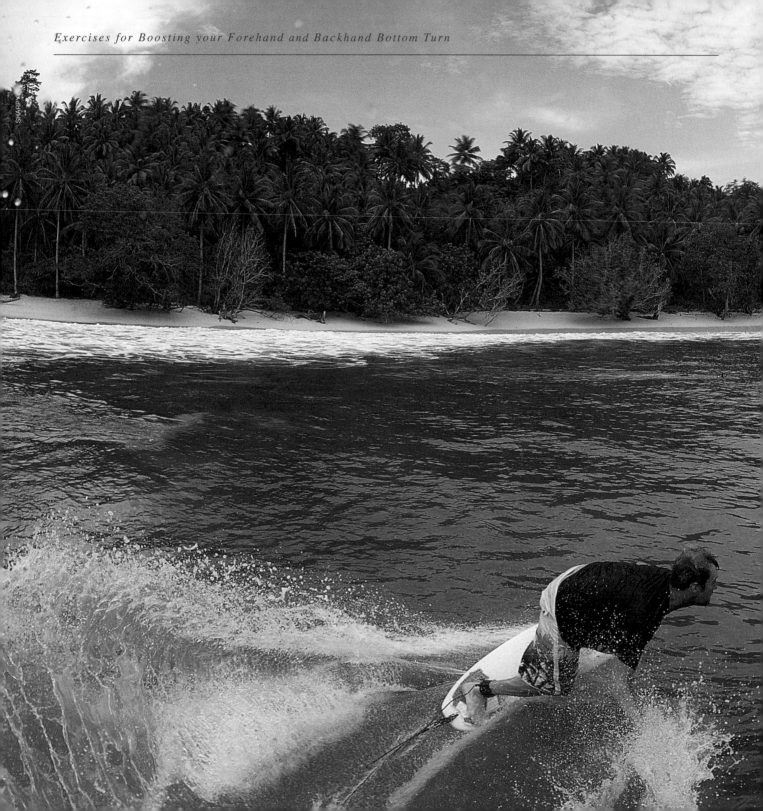

IF IT'S NOT CHALLENGING YOU, THEN IT'S NOT CHANGING YOU

HAMSTRINGS & GLUTEUS
MAXIMUS EXERCISES

As you drive up the lip of a wave your glutes (buttocks) aid in the movement. As you then begin to lean back into the next movement your legs work alongside your core, allowing you to remain in contact with the board.

BASIC SQUATS - BEGINNERS

Start the exercise by standing with your feet a hip width apart, keeping your shoulders back and arms out in front of you. Try using a chair for an improvement in your movement.

Stand with your legs against the chair, then just before your buttocks reach the chair stand up, this will allow a good 90 degree angle to take place in your legs.

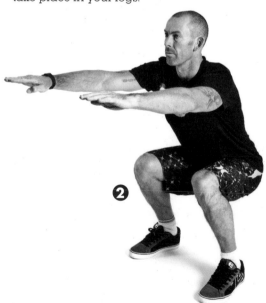

INDO BOARD SQUATS - INTERMEDIATE

Indo Boards are great for improving your leg strength. Stand on the deck with feet shoulder width apart, tilt pelvis back and bring hips back as you squat. Try not to let your knees get in front of your feet on the way down.

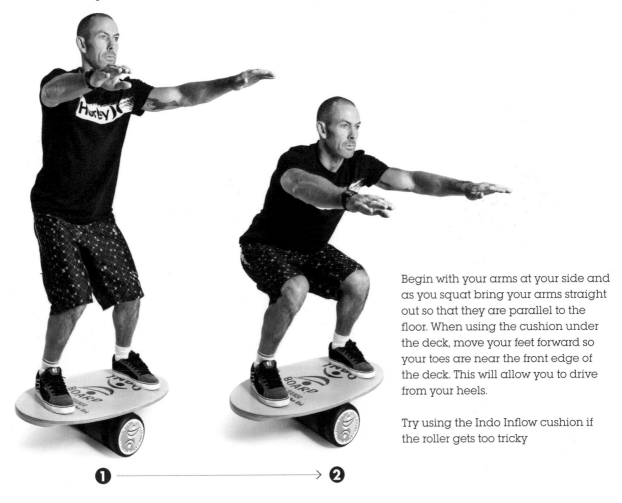

① ·········→ **②**

Begin with your arms at your side and as you squat bring your arms straight out so that they are parallel to the floor. When using the cushion under the deck, move your feet forward so your toes are near the front edge of the deck. This will allow you to drive from your heels.

Try using the Indo Inflow cushion if the roller gets too tricky

DYNAMIC EXERCISES

INDO TORSO TWISTS WITH ROLLER - BEGINNERS

Start the exercise by holding a back foot squat, then slowly stand up and swing your arms over the opposite shoulder – take care here to maintain a good centre of balance and then returning to the start position. After a twist, return to the start position.

① ··········▶ **②** ··········▶ **③**

INDO TORSO TWISTS WITH WEIGHT - INTERMEDIATE

Again start this exercise in the squat position. This time though, hold a light weight with both hands and from this position start to stand up and take the weight over your shoulder on your opposite side – take care here to maintain a good centre of balance. Your aim is to follow the weight directly behind you while your lower body points forwards.

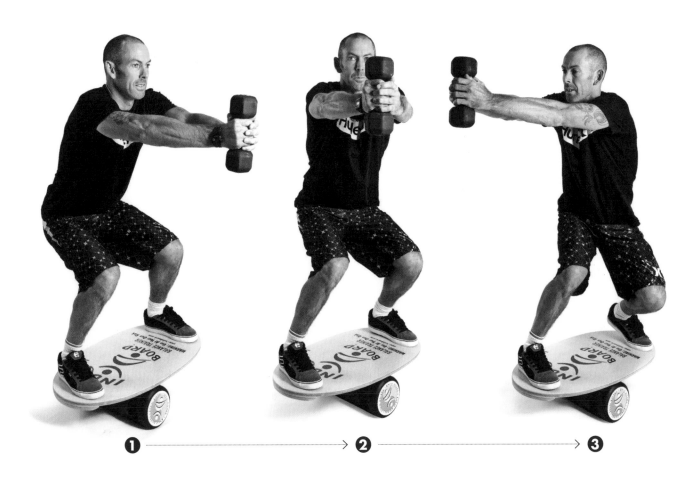

① → ② → ③

INDO TWISTS WITH WEIGHT - ADVANCED

To advance the move to its max simply speed things up. Maintain a good centre of balance and you may want to build up your speed on each rep.

INDO BOARD SQUATS WITH
MEDICINE BALL TWISTS - ADVANCED

Start this exercise in the same way as the basic squat. This time there will be a lot more balance involved – which will mimic the movements of the bottom turn and overload the muscle groups involved.

Start with the ball positioned on one side of you, and as you come upwards from a squat stand up and twist. Repeat this move 5 times on each side. As you get stronger and your balance improves increase the reps.

This can also be done on a BOSU Balance Trainer.

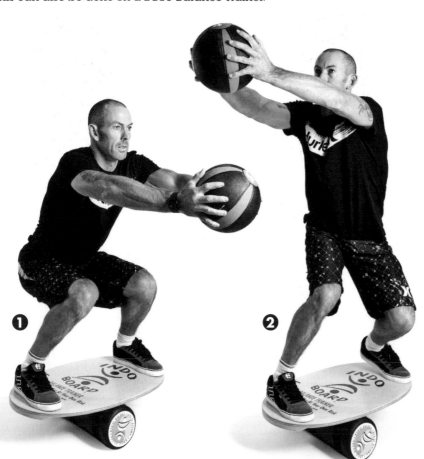
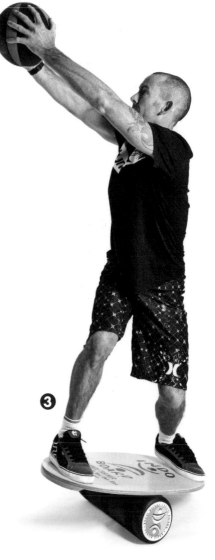

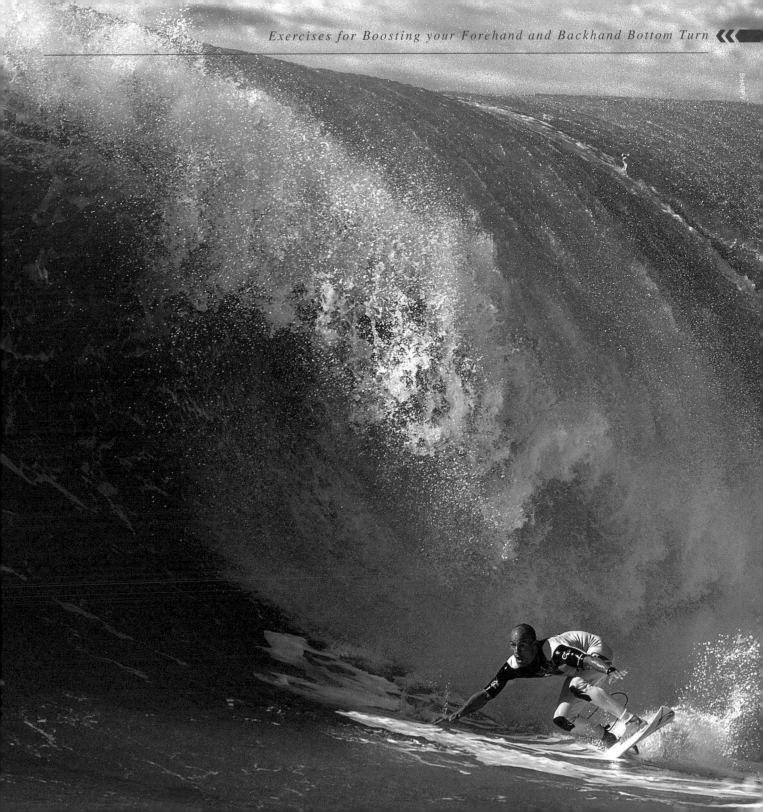

SNAPS OFF THE LIP

The snap is not a cutback. It's a quick directional change and can be as demanding as you make it.

It's a great move when you're first learning to turn because you don't have to set your rail perfectly, however there is more demand on the body the faster you move. It's also a perfect set up move for an experienced surfer who's flowing into a big combo or hitting an air section. Strength and stamina play a key role in just how well you do this.

Good joint stabilisation and body position on the board is very important. Good ankle and knee stability can increase speed and power through the movement – any exercises done should reflect this.

Balance training can help this movement to become more powerful and can make a real difference if mixed with repetitive sets of exercises.

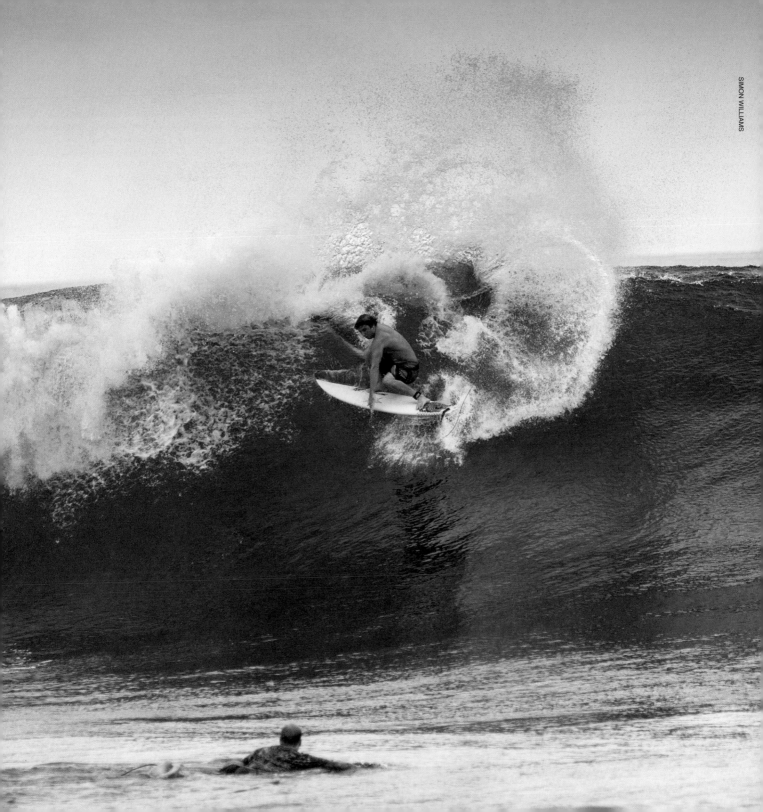

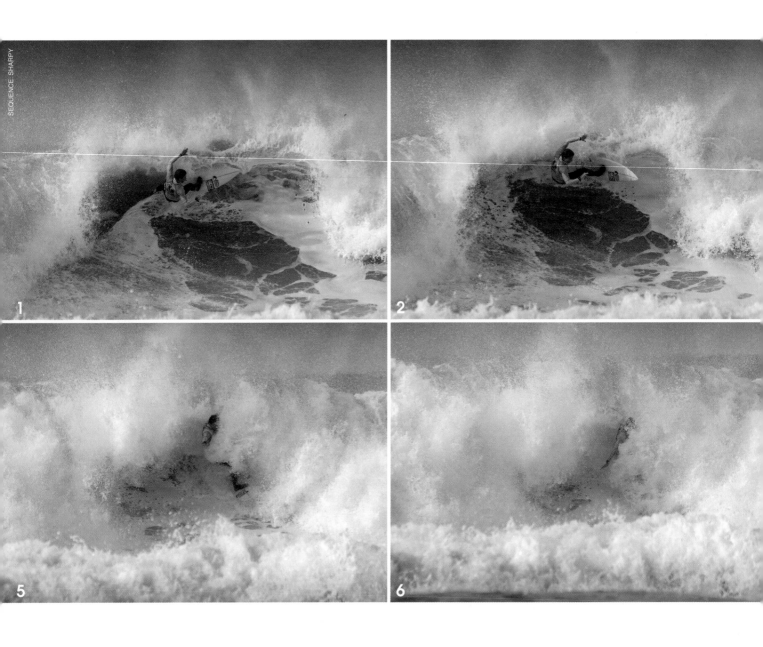

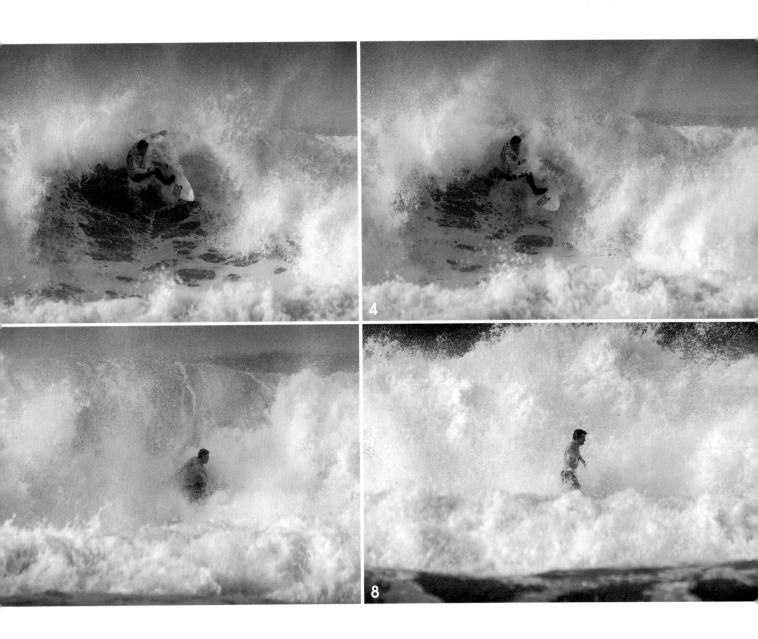

CORE EXERCISES

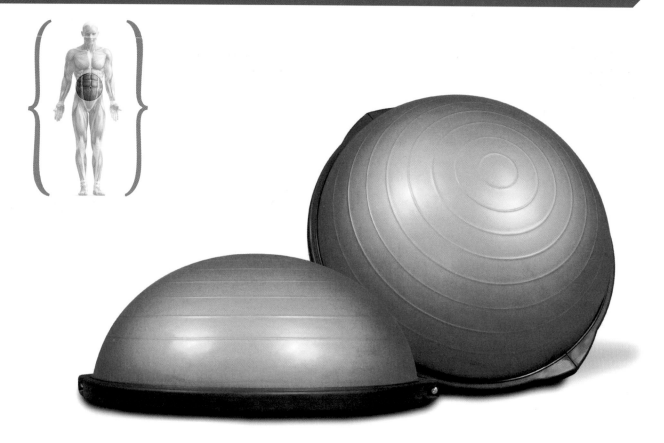

[THE BOSU CAN BE USED FOR: SPORTS CONDITIONING (BOTH AEROBIC & ANAEROBIC), STABILISATION, AGILITY TRAINING, STABILITY AND FLEXIBILITY TRAINING FOR THE TRUNK, AND STRENGTH TRAINING FOR THE ENTIRE BODY.]

BOSU PLANK - BEGINNERS

Grab each side of the Bosu Balance Trainer with the dome side down. Keep your head in line with the spine, your back straight, and feet slightly apart, then hold.

Hold this position for as long as you can, engage your core, and keep the tummy tight.

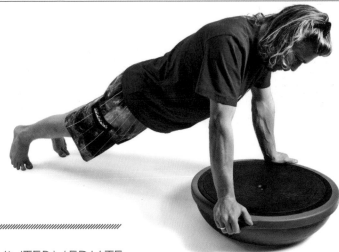

BOSU PLANK WITH LEG RAISE - INTERMEDIATE

It's simple to make this exercise harder; simply hold your position and, while doing so, lift one foot off the floor a few inches. Repeat this as many times as possible before resting.

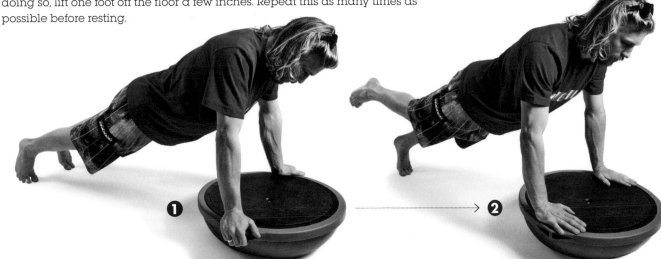

BOSU PLANK WITH LEG RAISE AND PRESS UP - ADVANCED

This exercise will really test your core. Start the exercise in the same way as before, then tilt the deck forwards and backwards four times. Maintain a good, safe body position while doing this.

Once you've completed four tilts, do one press up, and then repeat the whole process until you reach exhaustion.

OBLIQUES EXERCISES

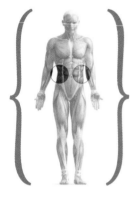

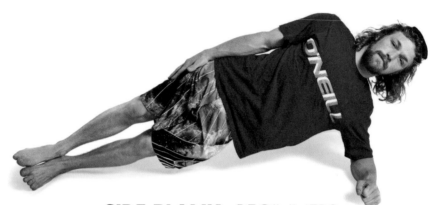

SIDE PLANK - BEGINNERS

Start this exercise by resting on one arm, keeping your upper body in line with your lower body, your head in line with your spine, and one leg on top of the other. Hold for around 10-15 seconds before changing sides.

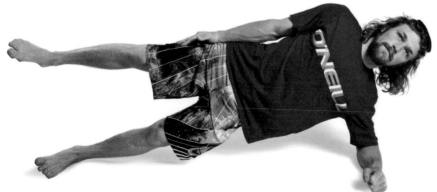

SIDE PLANK WITH LEG RAISE - INTERMEDIATE

Begin this exercise in the same way as the beginners side plank. Once you have a good body position, lift one leg off the other for around 3-4 seconds. Try this several times before changing sides.

SIDE PLANK WITH WEIGHT - ADVANCED

Once you have built up a good base of strength you may wish to try an advanced side plank. For this you can either use some ankle weights or hand weight. As with the intermediate side plank, lift one leg off the other for around 3-5 seconds.

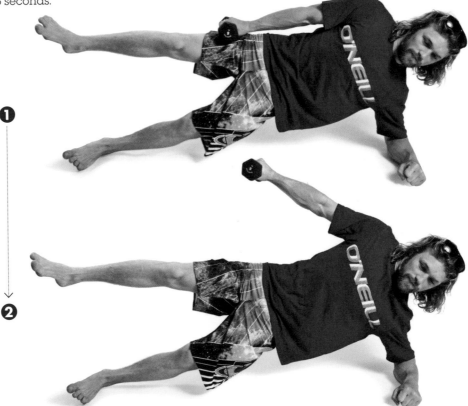

①

②

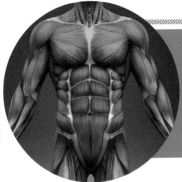

DECADE3D/SHUTTERSTOCK.COM

OBLIQUE AND CORE STABILITY TRAINING

THE AIM OF CORE STRENGTH TRAINING IS TO INCREASE THE EFFICIENCY OF THE SMALLER, DEEPER, STABILISING MUSCLES WHICH HELP YOU BALANCE, SUCH AS THE OBLIQUES AND TRANSVERSE ABDOMINALS WHICH LIE DEEP WITHIN YOUR ABDOMINAL AREA.

KNEE AND ANKLE
STRENGTH

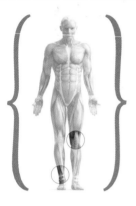

BOSU SINGLE LEG BALANCE
- BEGINNERS

To strengthen your ankles and knees try standing on the Bosu Balance Trainer with the dome side down.

Stand in the centre of the deck and raise one foot slightly off the deck whilst maintaining a good upright body posture.

Hold for 8-10 seconds before changing legs.

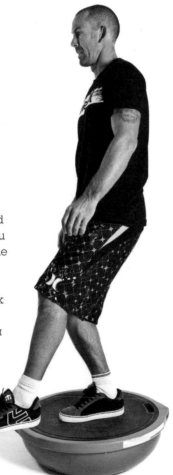

KNEE TIPS

THE BEST WAY TO PREVENT INJURY IS TO MAINTAIN STRONG KNEES AND ANKLES. SURFING HAS MANY DIVERSE MOVEMENTS AND THEY ALL PUT DEMANDS ON THE KNEES AND ANKLES AS YOU TRANSFER BALANCE DURING THE MOVEMENTS.

KNEE LIGAMENTS CAN GET STRETCHED (SPRAINED), OR SOMETIMES TORN BADLY (RUPTURED). A LIGAMENT RUPTURE CAN BE PARTIAL (JUST SOME OF THE FIBRES THAT MAKE UP THE LIGAMENT ARE TORN) OR COMPLETE (THE LIGAMENT IS TORN THROUGH COMPLETELY). THIS IS THE WORST KIND OF KNEE INJURY AND CAN PUT A SURFER OUT FOR MONTHS, SO KEEP DOING THESE EXERCISES TO PREVENT INJURY TO YOUR KNEES AND ANKLES.

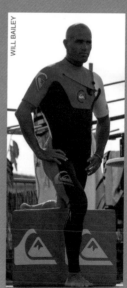

WILL BAILEY

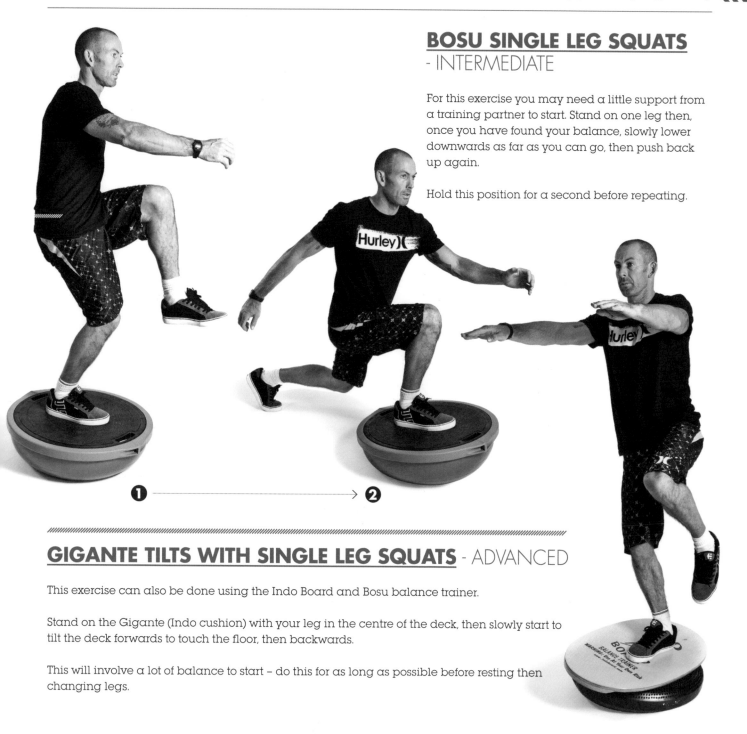

BOSU SINGLE LEG SQUATS
- INTERMEDIATE

For this exercise you may need a little support from a training partner to start. Stand on one leg then, once you have found your balance, slowly lower downwards as far as you can go, then push back up again.

Hold this position for a second before repeating.

❶ ------------------------------→ ❷

GIGANTE TILTS WITH SINGLE LEG SQUATS - ADVANCED

This exercise can also be done using the Indo Board and Bosu balance trainer.

Stand on the Gigante (Indo cushion) with your leg in the centre of the deck, then slowly start to tilt the deck forwards to touch the floor, then backwards.

This will involve a lot of balance to start – do this for as long as possible before resting then changing legs.

LEG STRENGTH

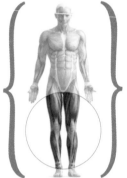

As you drive up the lip of a wave your glutes (buttocks) aid in the movement. As you then begin to lean back into the next movement your legs work alongside your core, allowing you to remain in contact with the board.

REVERSE LUNGES
- BEGINNERS

Although the basic lunge (in a forwards movement) is highly beneficial for boosting your surfing leg power, it is really important not to overdo the amount of lunges that you do. Reverse lunges, however, have less of an impact on the knee.

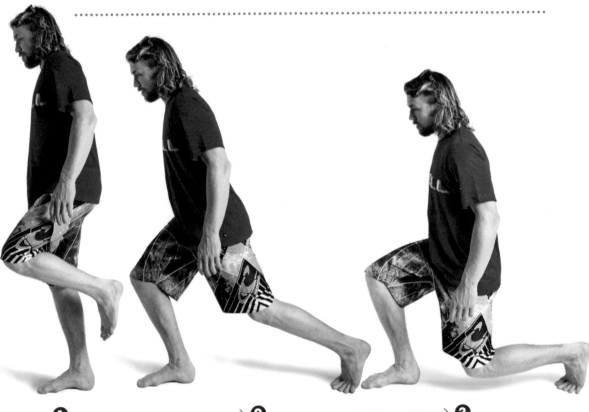

①   **②**   **③**

To start the exercise stand with hands on hips, shoulders back. From this position step backwards and lunge to about 90 degrees before repeating the move on the other side.

REVERSE LUNGE WITH WEIGHTS - INTERMEDIATE

This exercise is basically the same move as before, only this time you will hold light weights in your hands for added resistance; again keep your shoulders back through the move and maintain good technique.

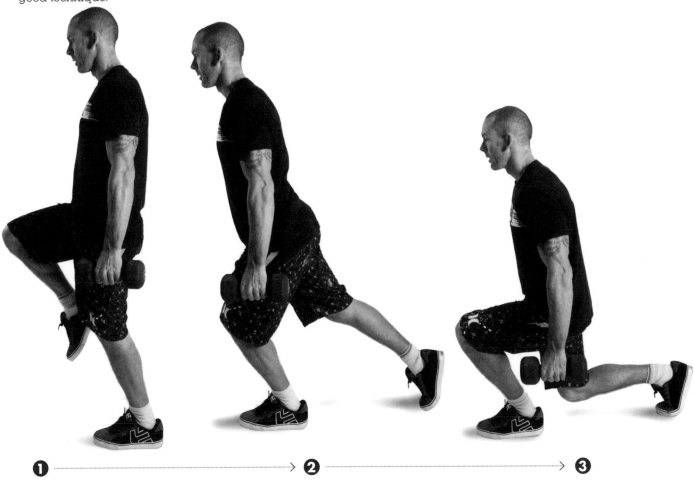

❶ ....> ❷ ....> ❸

REVERSE LUNGE INTO FORWARDS LUNGE - ADVANCED

Start the exercise by lunging backwards, then go straight into a forwards lunge. Maintain a good technique and posture before repeating. For added resistance use weights.

BALANCE AND
PROPRIOCEPTION SKILLS

Cracking your board off the lip can be as demanding as you make it. At any level this requires balance and proprioception skill. In many surfing movements you won't always have eye contact with your board, and this is where training in this area can help.

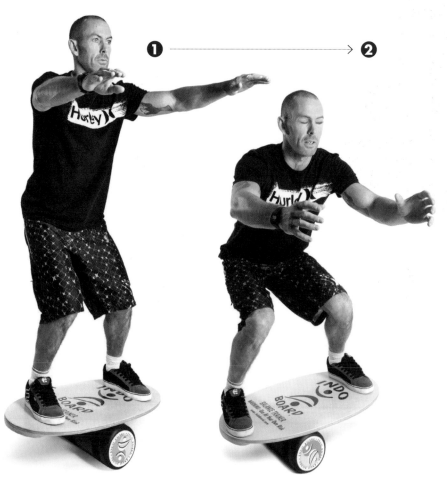

❶ ....➤ **❷**

INDO SQUAT
WITH EYES CLOSED
- BEGINNERS

Try standing on your Indo Board with feet about a hip width apart, knees slightly bent, then once you feel stable try closing your eyes.

Closing your eyes will heighten your proprioceptive skills. (This exercise is best done using a partner for safety!)

BOSU MEDICINE BALL SQUATS WITH THROW OVER - INTERMEDIATE

Start the exercise by standing with your feet a hip width apart on the deck, then slowly squat downwards into a basic squat position with arms out in front.

Then take a medicine ball from your feet and over your opposite shoulder. Try a series of different directions for best results. Remember to maintain a centre of balance in the same way you would on your board.

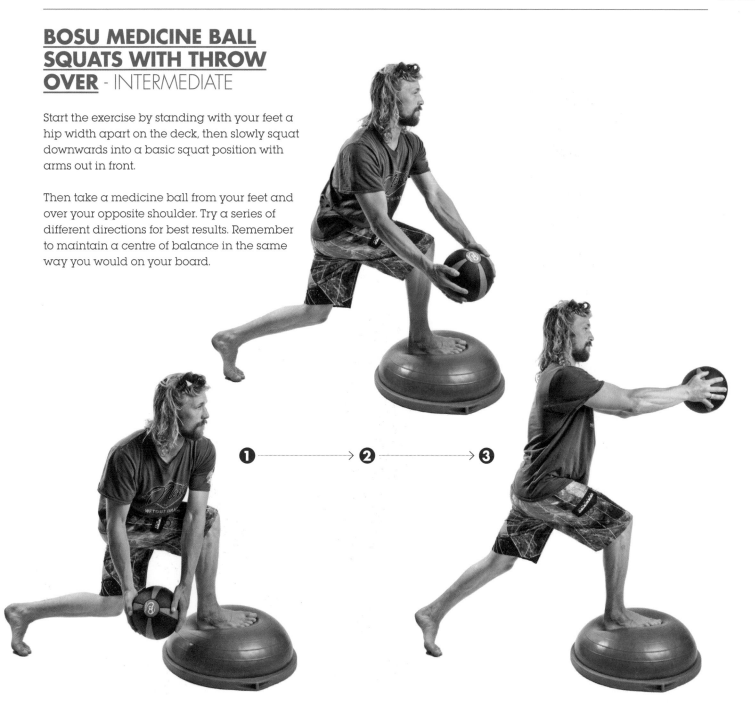

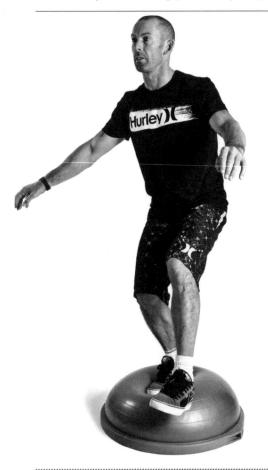

LUNGE TO SINGLE LEG BALANCE WITH BOSU BALANCE TRAINER - ADVANCED

Before attempting this move make sure you have a good level of fitness and strength; you will need to turn the dome side up.

Start the exercise in the same way as a normal lunge, only this time place the leading foot in the centre of the upturned Bosu deck. (Note: this will be very unstable.)

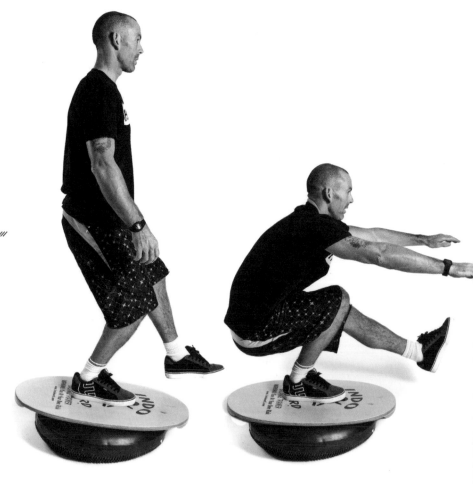

SINGLE LEG SQUAT ON GIGANTE AND INDO BOARD - ADVANCED

Standing on the centre of the deck with one leg slightly bent, slowly squat down with the other leg stetched to the front.

Remember this is an advanced exerscie so take care. You may need a training partner to help getting back up if you're not strong enough!

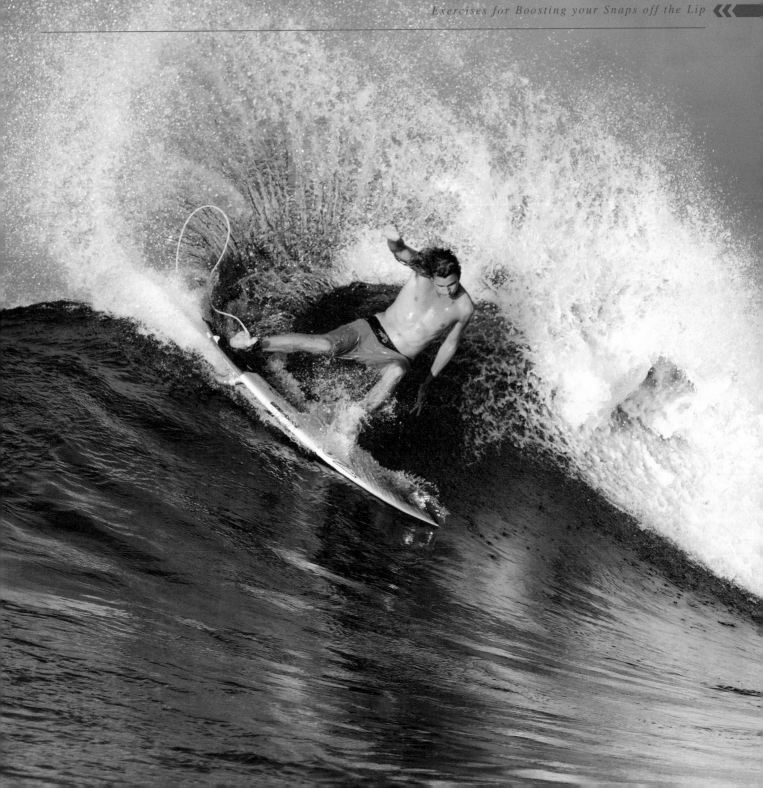

DYNAMIC POWER
EXERCISES

LUNGE TO SINGLE LEG BALANCE
- BEGINNERS

Start the exercise in a 90 degree lunge position then, maintaining your balance, quickly bring the extended leg forwards so that your knee comes upwards to your chest.

Tighten your core for stability and hold, and then repeat.

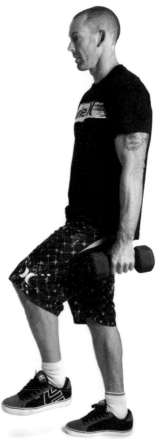
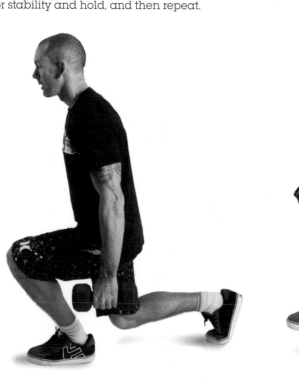

① ----------> **②**

LUNGE TO SINGLE LEG BALANCE
WITH MEDICINE BALL - INTERMEDIATE

This time add a medicine ball for added resistance. Start the move with the ball down on the floor, then once you're ready explode upwards bringing your knee upwards again as you throw to follow your knee.

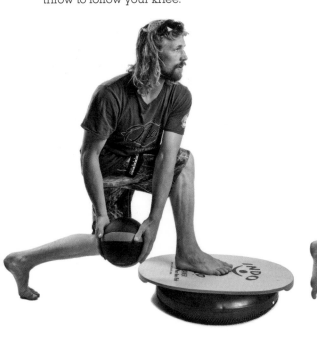
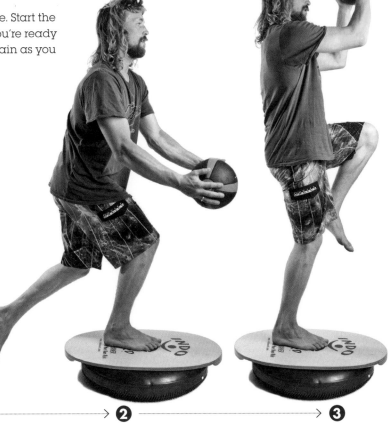

1 ··········> **2** ··········> **3**

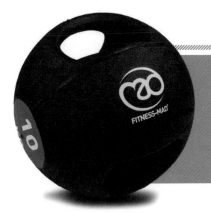

MEDICINE BALL EXERCISES FOR SURFING

ORIGINATING FROM PERSIA OVER 3000 YEARS AGO, MEDICINE BALL EXERCISES ARE GREAT FOR IMPROVING FORCE PRODUCTION AND REINFORCING STABILITY WITHIN SPECIFIC PLANES OF MOVEMENT. USING A MEDICINE BALL TO TRAIN THE CORE IS PERFECT BECAUSE YOU CAN PERFORM MANY FUNCTIONAL MOVEMENTS SIMILAR TO THOSE USED WHEN SURFING.

ENHANCE YOUR BARREL RIDING

If you're looking to enhance your barrel riding experience, then speed and agility are the key. The fact is that getting barrelled properly takes a lot of skill, but training is also essential. There's no exercise in the world to mimic the actual dynamics of barrel riding, but you can help along the way with some basic exercises.

The challenge of barrel riding is finding enough speed of movement, combined with the correct timing – very often all within a split second of dropping into a wave. With all this in mind any exercise should be done fast!

Any training you do should really involve explosive movements, i.e. plyometrics (dynamic movements that improve your body's movement and alertness).

There is a very simple exercise that most of us have done at school: the squat thrust. This will improve your dynamic leg speed (i.e. quicker pop up) into that secure position for hitting your line.

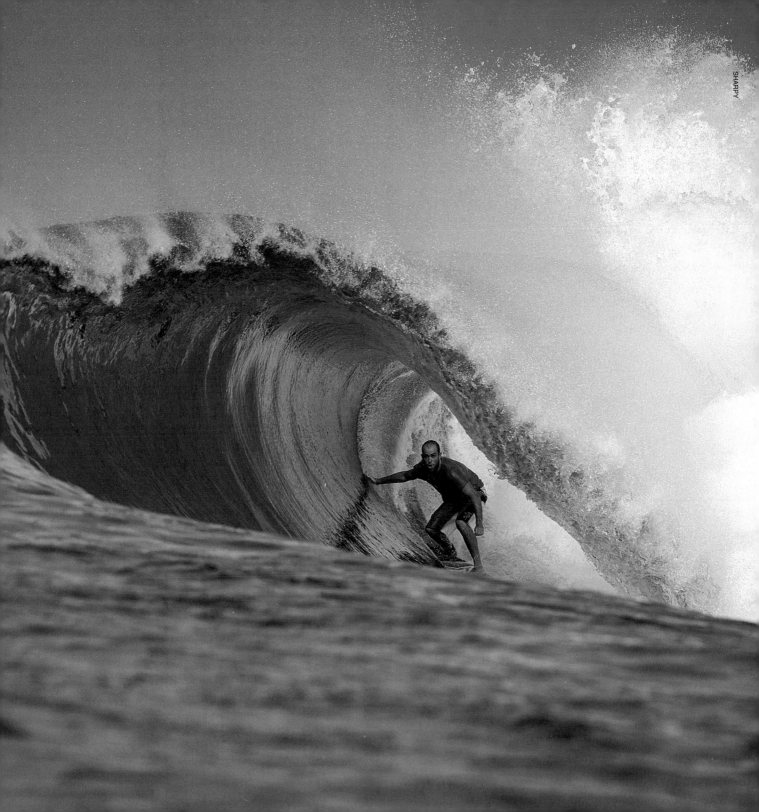

001
SQUAT THRUSTS

Start the exercise in the press up position, hands in line with your shoulders.

Bring the knees forwards at speed, feet together, then quickly extend the legs back to the starting position. Repeat this 5 times before resting.

As you get stronger you may wish to increase the reps. Try building up to 6x15 reps and do this at least once or twice a week to see improved results in your pop ups. You can also add a jump up at the each of each squat thrust.

Doing squat thrusts isn't going to be enough on its own. To improve your surf fitness you will need to incorporate them into a well balanced training programme.

In addition to dynamic leg movements, getting barrelled takes a heightened level of proprioceptive skill (balance). Any balance kit that will allow you to fine tune your backhand can be highly useful.

The Indo board has been around for years. It really can be a great bit of kit. Now with the introduction of the Indo Flo Gigante, you can practice your backhand or forehand over and over again.

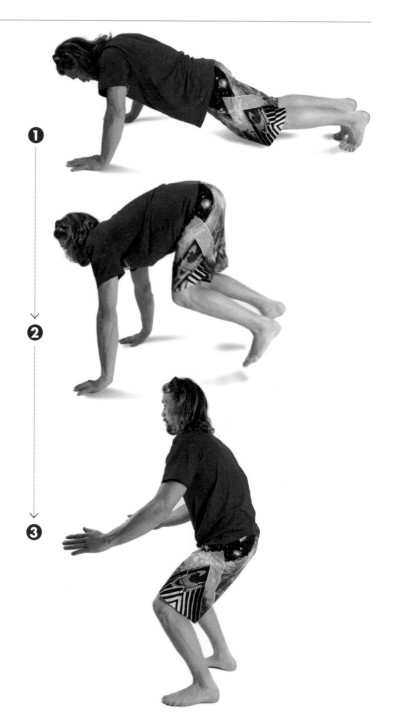

002
INDO ROLLER BACK HAND SQUATS
Boosts Leg Strength and Barrel Riding Balance.

This can also be done with the Gigante which can add extra stability to the move.

Start the exercise in the backhand position. Hold this for 3 seconds then stand up (but not fully, about 95%). Then slowly drop down again into your backhand position.

Do this 5 times, rest then repeat. This will strengthen your legs and aid your backhand balance big time.

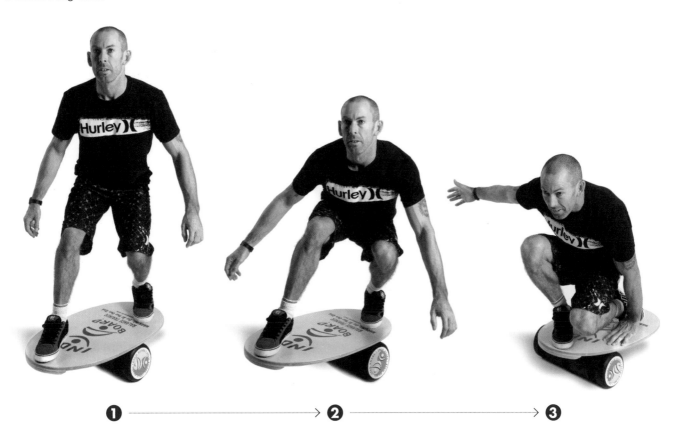

❶ ---------------------➤ ❷ ---------------------➤ ❸

003
INDO BOARD AND THE GIGANTE/BOSU
3 EXERCISES IN ONE.

This all in one blast of an exercise involves an Indo Board and the Indo Gigante. Or you can do the exercise without any kit to start with.

Start in the press up position with a straight back, hands in line with your shoulders, and tummy muscles/core tightened. The aim is to quickly bring both feet forwards at the same time onto the Indo Board, then up into a standing position, and then drop back down into a press up position and do a press up. Repeat the move 5 times.

This exercise will boost your pop up strength, core strength, speed, agility and explosive power all in one. All the factors involved in scoring that perfect barrel!

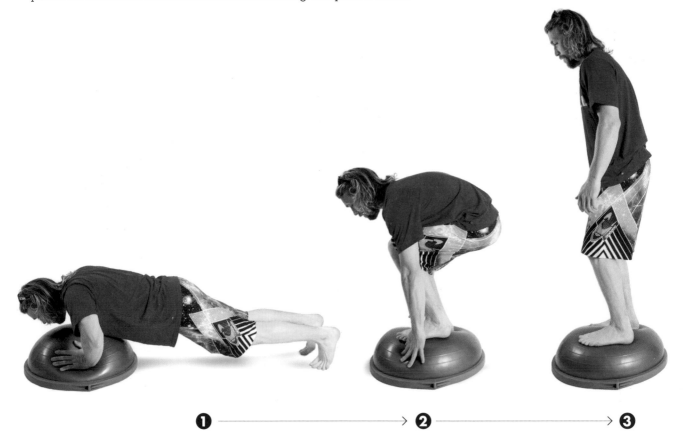

❶ ....➤ ❷ ....➤ ❸

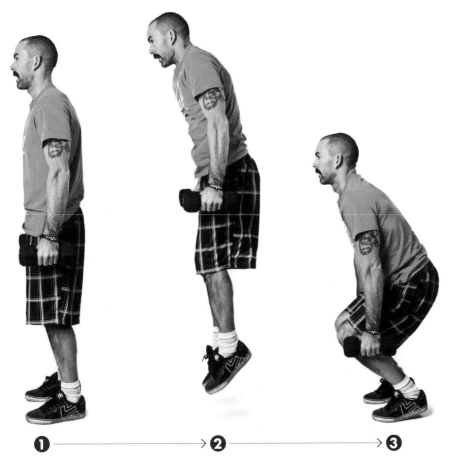

004
BURPEE WITH WEIGHTS

Says what it is – a burpee holding weights. This is a great exercise including all the factors involved in scoring that perfect barrel!

If you're new to it try it without weights first.

Start by standing with your back straight and weights by your sides.

From here jump upwards, then quickly down into a press up position, extend your legs really well, then reverse.

Repeat, 6-8 reps

① ....➔ **②** ....➔ **③**

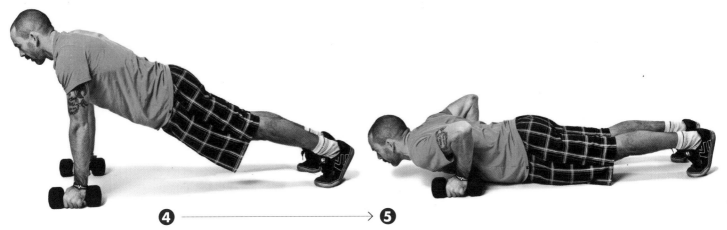

④ ....➔ **⑤**

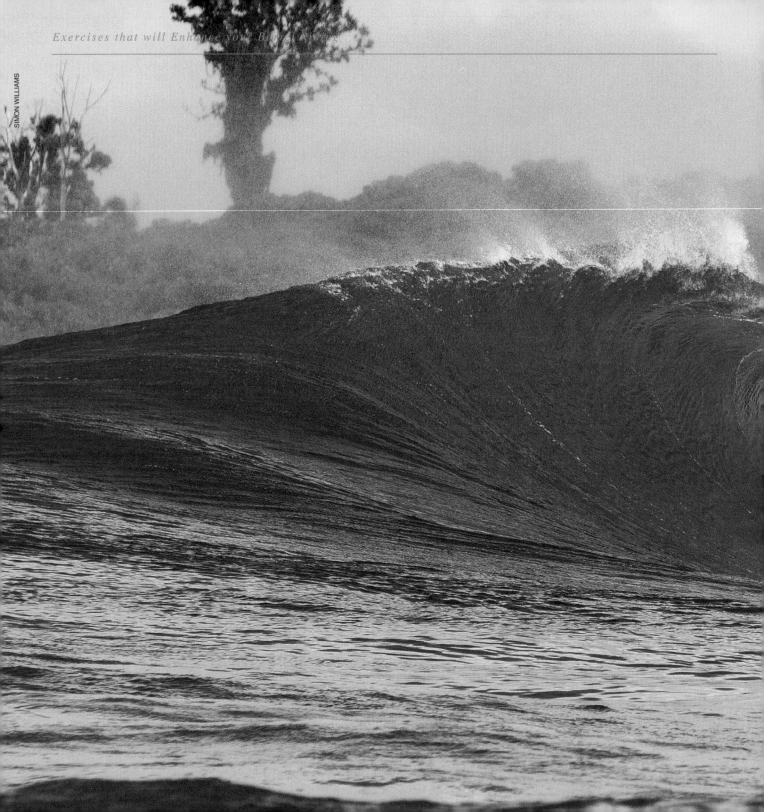

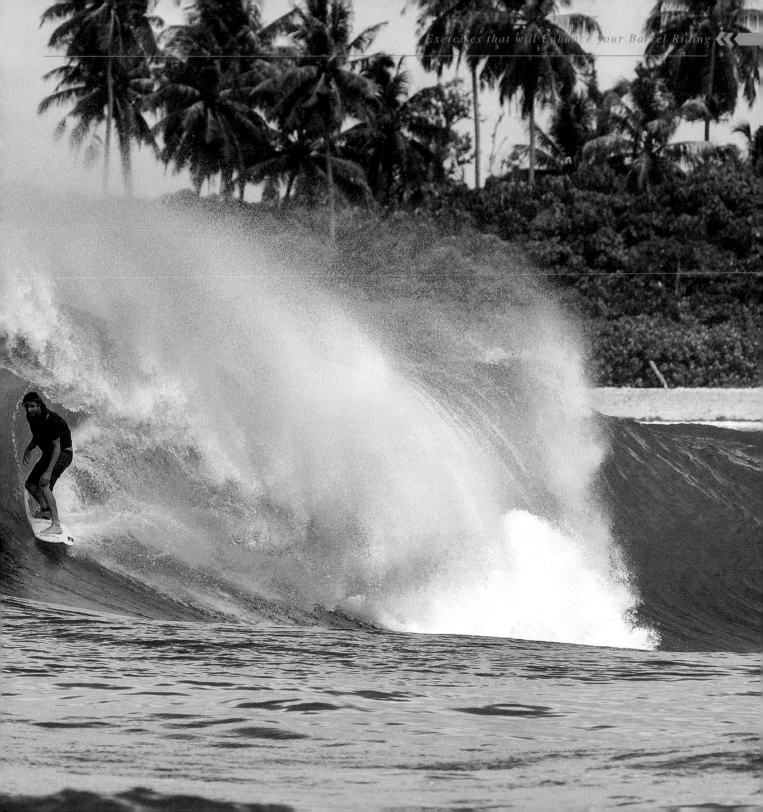

LAND TRAINING FOR BOOSTING AIRS

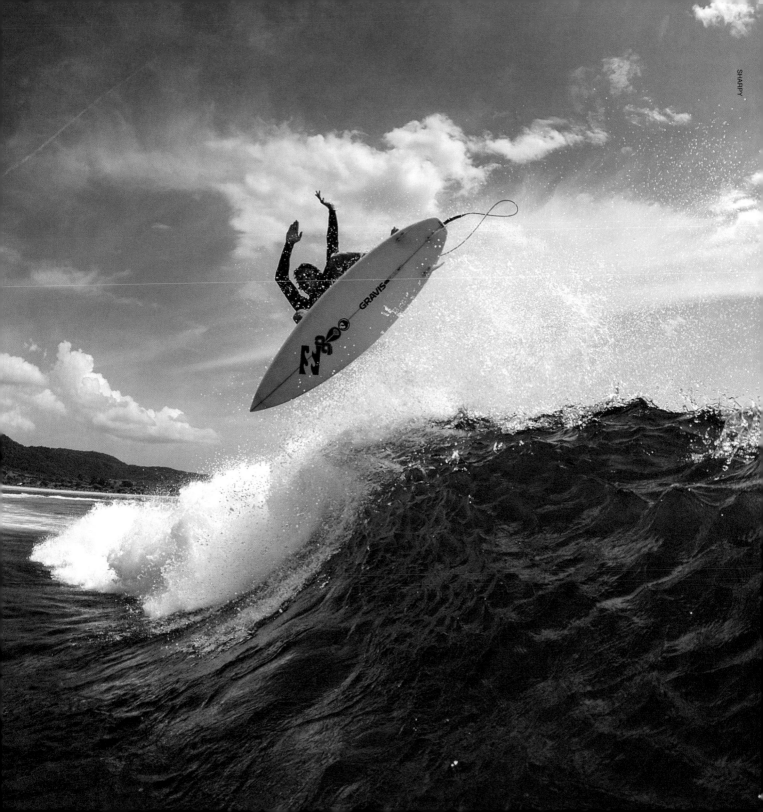

Many surfers dream of boosting an aerial surfing manoeuvre and landing it with ease, but modern day surfing seems to be advancing so much that it is now the norm to boost airs.

The fact is though, that this type of surfing may be for the few that have an inner ability to read their body's movements and the wave so accurately. However, with additional balance training, the use of the trampoline and some strength training, it is possible to improve your aerial potential.

An important factor to take into consideration is age. If you are now approaching middle age then your development in this area is going to be affected! In addition to age, proprioception skills (also known as the sixth sense) will play a major roll. Proprioception is the regulatory system of the body that governs the ability to generate and maintain an effective upright posture and physical balance – key factors in boosting airs.

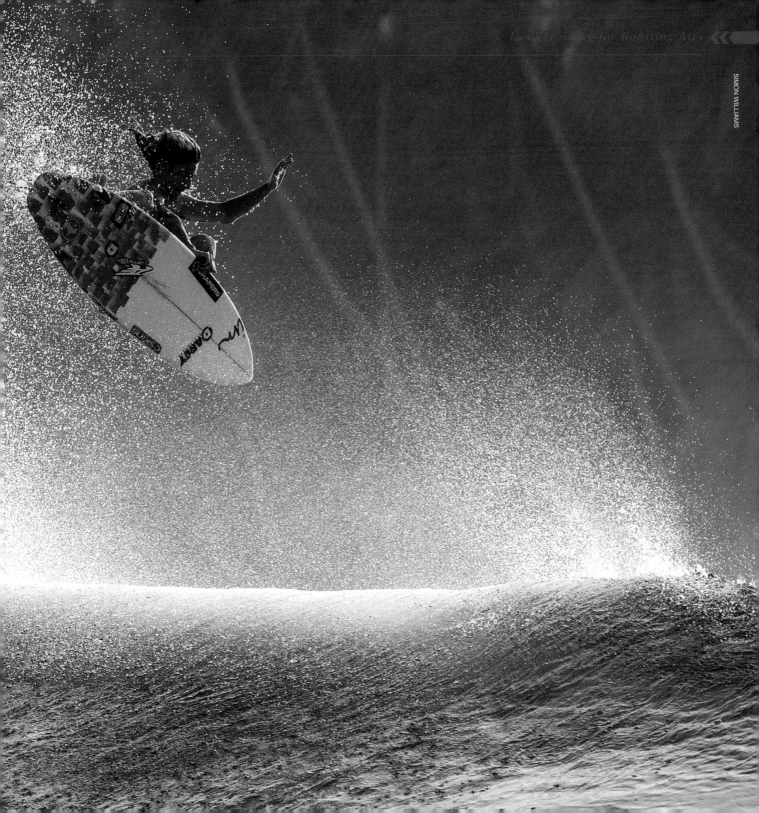

SIMON WILLIAMS

SIMPLE MULTI DIRECTIONAL
JUMPING MOVEMENTS

This may seem an odd way to improve your aerial acrobatics, but training your body to move in this way will improve your skills for landing.

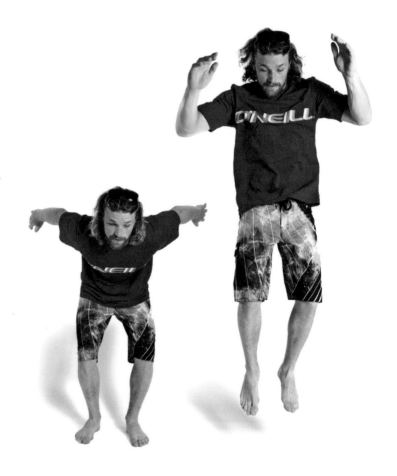

FORWARDS TO SIDEWARDS
JUMP - BEGINNERS

Start by facing forwards, feet slightly apart, and quickly jump forwards then sidewards. Freeze before repeating. The sidewards turning movement takes place in mid flight.

FORWARDS TO SIDEWARDS
THEN TWIST - INTERMEDIATE

Start this move with the same position as the last, then jump forwards. After this very quickly jump and turn 180 degrees, stick and freeze. Do this 4-5 times. You may wish to adapt this movement slightly while on the trampoline.

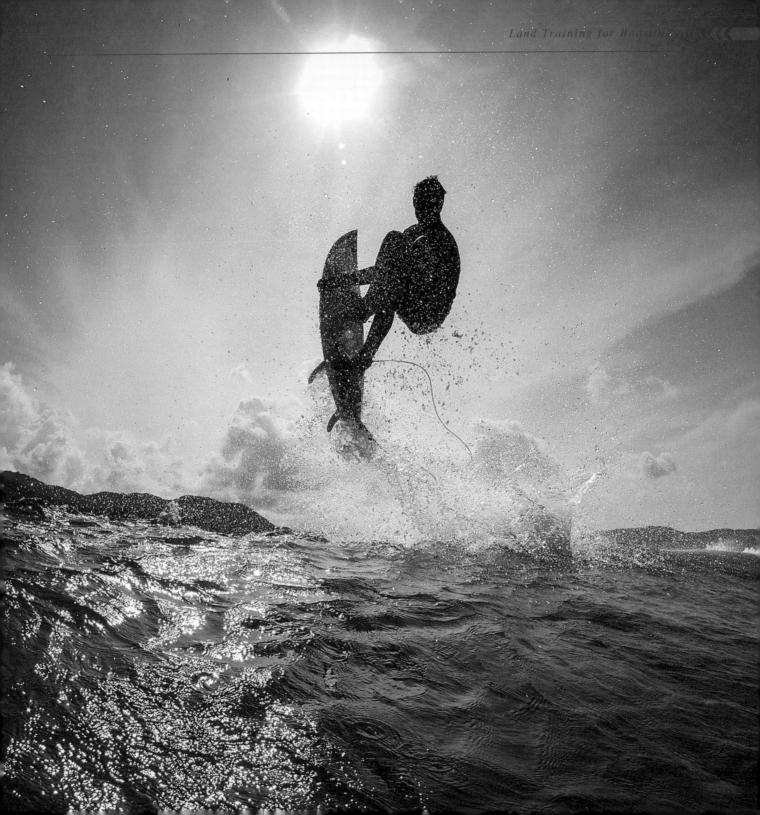

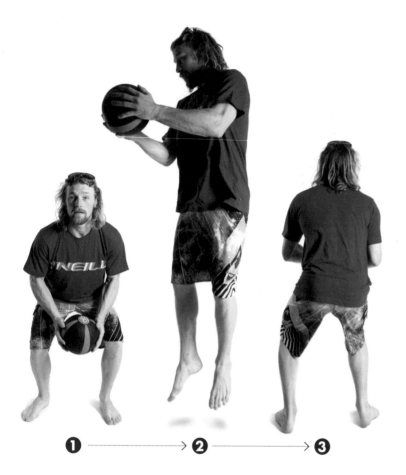

① -----> **②** -----> **③**

SPIN AND SQUAT
- ADVANCED
Warning this move will make you dizzy!

Start this exercise with both feet pointing forwards, legs slightly bent, arms slightly out to the side, then in one move jump and spin 180 degrees back to your starting position.

REVERSE BACKWARDS JUMP WITH MEDICINE BALL
- ADVANCED
Warning this move will make you dizzy!

Start the move with a medicine ball out in front of you with your legs apart, then jumping backwards quickly twist to face the other way.

As you jump backwards and rotate throw the medicine ball over your shoulder, staying in contact with the ball. Rest then jump again, only this time jump round so that you are facing forwards. At first you may need lots of rest before performing the move.

Practicing this type of multi directional and disorientating training will improve your ability to know where you are in relation to the wave during your flight over the wave.

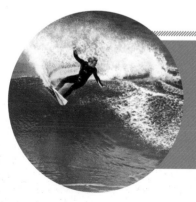

TRAIN REGULARLY TO REAP THE REWARDS

THE BENEFITS OF PLYOMETRICS ON SURFING CAN BE GREAT. HOWEVER THEY CAN BE GREATLY REDUCED UNLESS YOU TRAIN AT LEAST ONCE A WEEK AND BASIC PROGRESSION TAKES PLACE. FOR MAJOR IMPROVEMENTS IN EXPLOSIVE POWER I RECOMMEND TWO OR THREE 20-30 MINUTE WORKOUTS A WEEK AS A GOOD START.

BOSU TWIST AND STICK WITH OPTIONAL WEIGHT/MEDICINE BALL - ADVANCED

Warning this move will make you dizzy!

Make certain your Bosu is fixed securely. Then find your balance, soft knees, small jumps to start with then from there aim for larger twists. Once you have found a good rhythm repeat, but stop if you feel dizzy

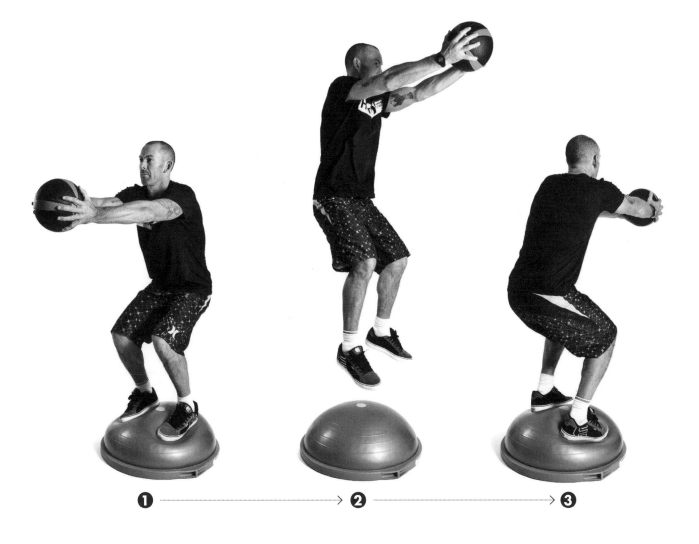

① ⟶ **②** ⟶ **③**

STRENGTHEN YOUR LANDING GEAR!

As you land your move, the higher the drop the more effort and strength will be needed. It's true to say that your knees will have to work hard to stabilise the drop, so strengthen the move with exercises that mimic the dropping phase of your manoeuvre.

DOUBLE LEG JUMPS IN A ROW - BEGINNERS

This exercise is best done on a soft surface: grass, sand, or with the use of a gym mat.

Start the exercise with both feet apart at about hip width, then simply jump forwards and land, directly after this repeat.

DOUBLE LEG JUMPS IN A ROW, WITH WEIGHTS - INTERMEDIATE

To advance this exercise simply add some free weights keeping them alongside your hips as you jump through the movements.

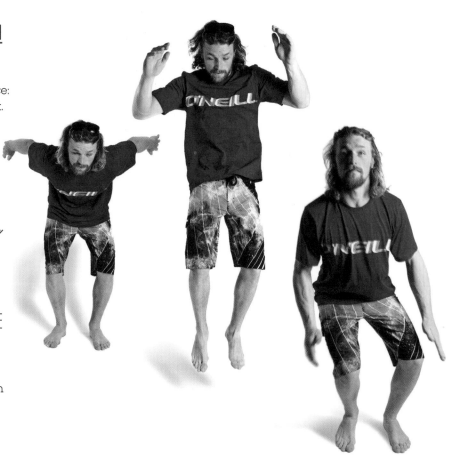

❶ ----------> ❷ ----------> ❸

INDO BOARD JUMP AND SQUAT
- ADVANCED

For this exercise you will need an Indo board and roller, or Gigante Inflow cushion.

Set your kit up a short distance away from you, bearing in mind that you will be jumping onto an unstable surface (you may wish to try this without the use of the Indo board before attempting the more advanced exercise).

Set yourself up into a press up position with both hands on the Indo deck, then with good focus explode forwards placing both feet on the deck holding a squat position. Rest, then repeat the move.

BOSU JUMP AND STICK WITH DUMBBELLS
- ADVANCED

The Bosu jump and stick is also a good exercise for improving the landing strength of your airs.

Set up the BOSU dome side up, then from a squat position and about half a meter away, jump and land with both feet. Keep the weights close to your body to add resistance during the move.

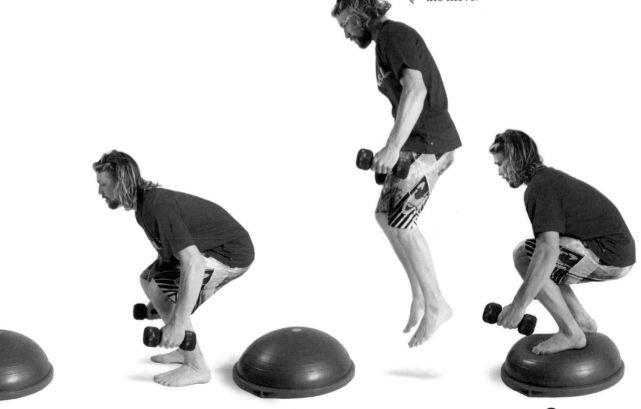

❶ -----> ❷ -----> ❸

TRAMPOLINE
EXERCISES

If you're lucky enough to have access to a trampoline then they can make a massive difference to your skill improvement; even basic exercises will help improve your air landing skills.

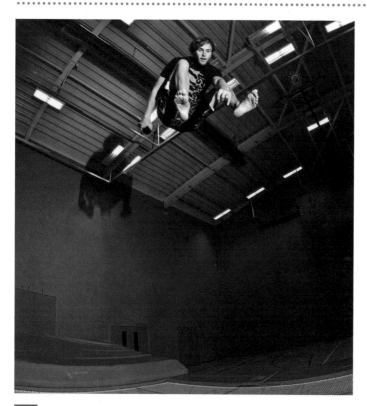

Being able to do airs may be for the few that have an inner ability to read their body's movements and the wave so accurately, but, with additional balance training, the use of a trampoline and some strength training it is possible to improve your airs.

By training on a trampoline you can improve your body's awareness to movement, which in turn will allow you to know where you are on your board in relation to the wave. Of course not everybody has access to a trampoline but using one will improve body awareness.

In addition to body awareness while boosting airs, it is also important to remember that what goes up must come down. The landing phase of any aerial surfing movement could well be the hardest part!

A surfer's ability to control the landing force after boosting an air will be dependent upon two factors: the general control of the body's momentum at landing and the ability of the surfer to dissipate the forces directed into the body to minimise impact upon the body.

[JUMPING AND LANDING EXERCISES CAN HELP IN THIS AREA; THEY WILL BOOST BODY AWARENESS AND MOVEMENT, IMPROVE BALANCE AND COORDINATION, AND BUILD STRENGTH IN THE LEGS.]

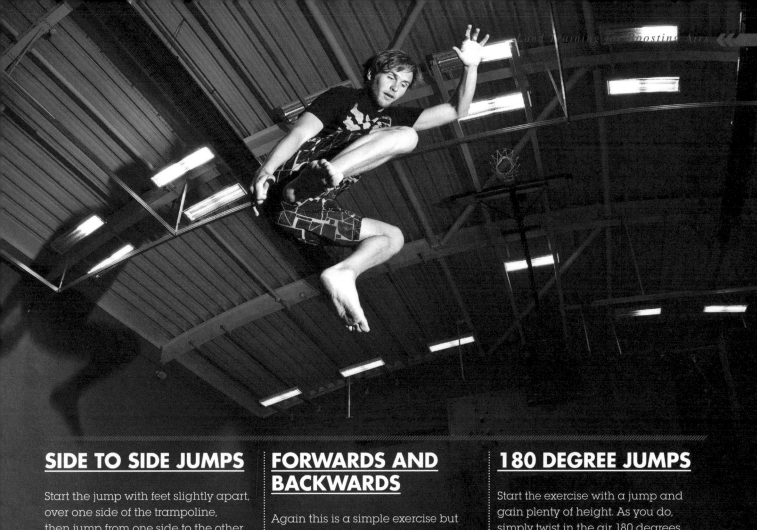

SIDE TO SIDE JUMPS

Start the jump with feet slightly apart, over one side of the trampoline, then jump from one side to the other, landing with soft knees to help stability and maintain a good posture, and keep the core tight.

FORWARDS AND BACKWARDS

Again this is a simple exercise but will allow you to build a good base for more advanced exercises on the trampoline. Soft knees and a tight core will allow for good stability.

180 DEGREE JUMPS

Start the exercise with a jump and gain plenty of height. As you do, simply twist in the air 180 degrees landing with both feet pointing in the opposite direction, rest and repeat.

SWIMMING FOR IMPROVED SURFING FITNESS

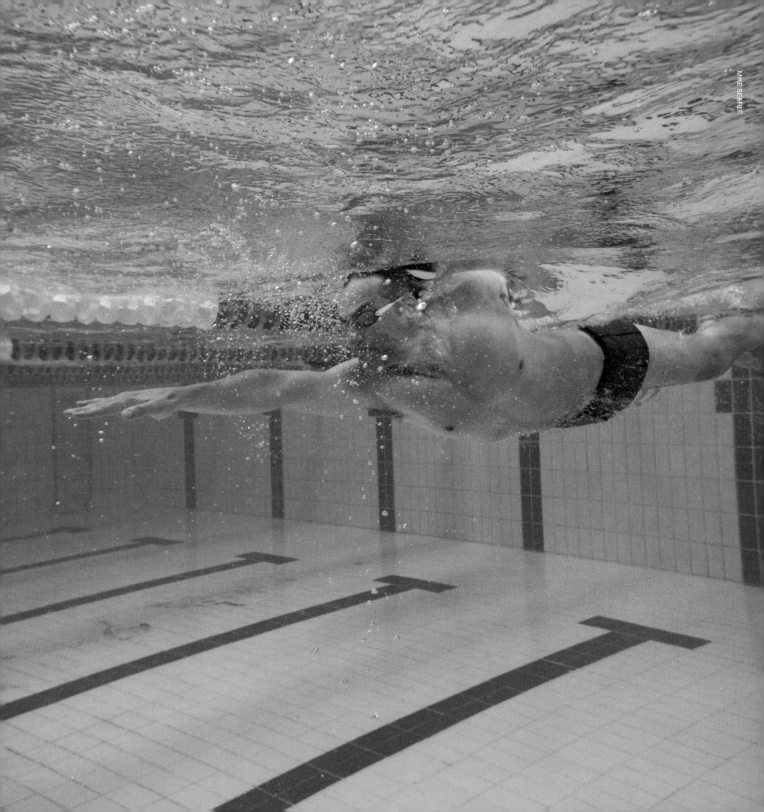

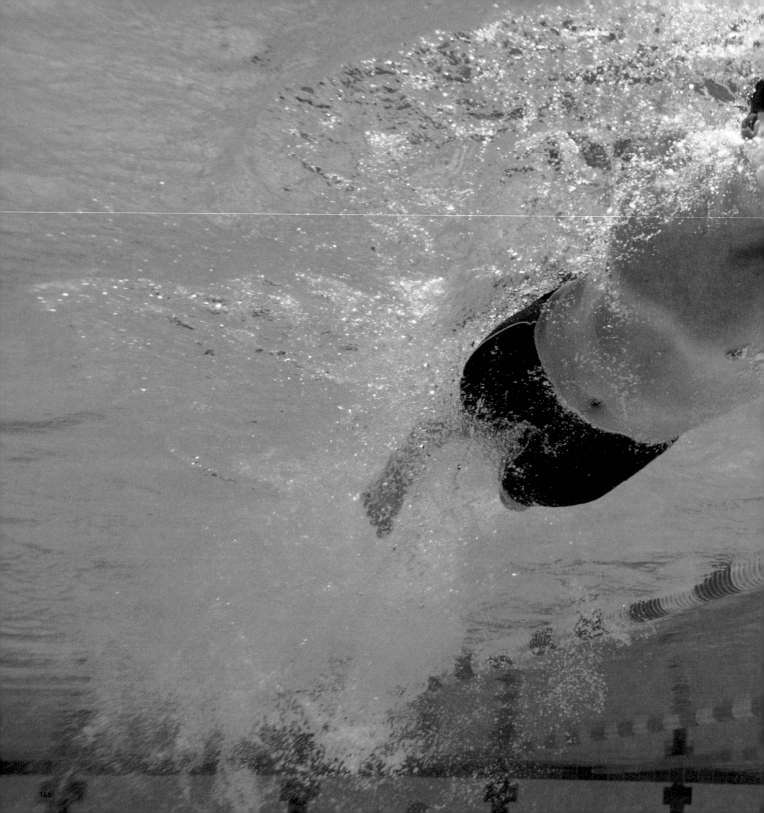

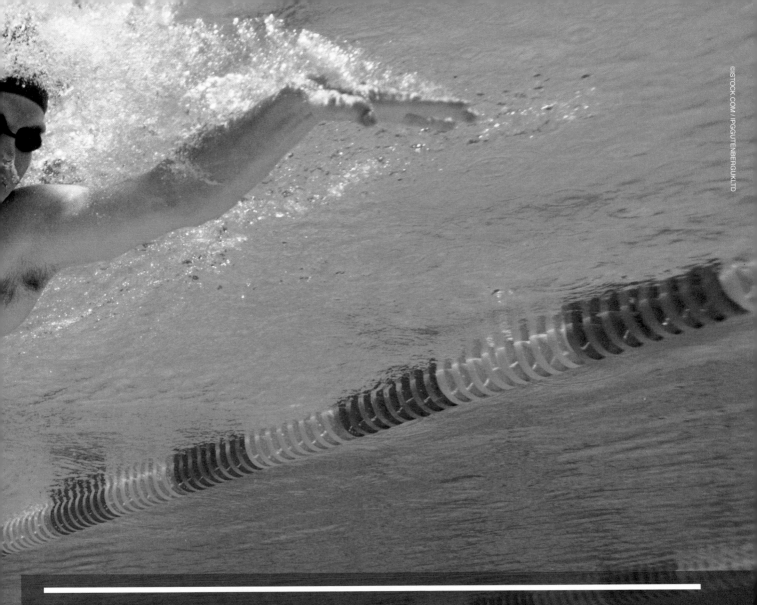

The simple fact is that swimming movements are so similar to surfing paddling movements, that a swim training programme is guaranteed to boost your surfing fitness. The arm movements and aerobic and anaerobic demands that surfing places on your body can be copied and applied in the swimming pool. Breath holding sets (hypoxic, without oxygen) and training can also be applied.

NB: if your swimming is not that good then seek additional help from a swimming coach or teacher.

No two surfing sessions are the same, so you should prepare your surfing fitness for all conditions. More strenuous sessions could be:

• Cross onshore surf making the paddle out longer, with more duck diving
• Big swell days
• Different times of tide creating different conditions in one session

On these more challenging days, the demands on your body are going to go up significantly and it takes many chemical changes within your body to allow you to perform. Or even just to get out back!

You may feel a burning sensation in your back and shoulders as your body breaks down Adenosine Triphosphate (ATP), via a procedure called anaerobic glycolysis – this is the breakdown of carbohydrates. The fitter you are the more oxygenated red blood cells you have in your body, which help to remove waste products from the body as energy is supplied.

Lactic acid is a term used most commonly by athletes to describe the intense pain felt during exhaustive or high levels of sprinting and exercise; however it is not the lactic acid that causes the pain, but the build up of Pyruvic Acid and Hydrogen ions or (H+). This process will be much more intense if the body has insufficient oxygen through lack of good physical condition. With improved physical condition there will be more available oxygen for the chemical processes in the body to work more efficiently. If your body is not in peak physical condition then the Hydrogen ions will not be removed into the body and will build up in the muscles. This can lead to muscle soreness and stiffness 1-2 days after an intense surfing session. Equally, it will slow you down as you try to duck dive and paddle out. If you find yourself stuck in a rippy situation these effects will intensify your difficulties, as do the presence of Hydrogen ions, which make the muscle more acidic and will eventually halt muscle function. This could take your heart rate up into anaerobic levels, which

are about 85-95% of your max heart rate: at this point breathing will be heavy as your body has to work harder.

JUST A FEW REASONS WHY SWIM TRAINING IS SO GOOD FOR SURFERS:

• Catch more fatter waves, and get into small, sloppy waves earlier
• Increase aerobic capacity for paddle outs
• Higher levels of fitness during any unforeseen moments, like leash snaps, or bad rips
• Higher levels of endurance for longer surfing sessions
• Fast paddle power to make it out past sneaker sets

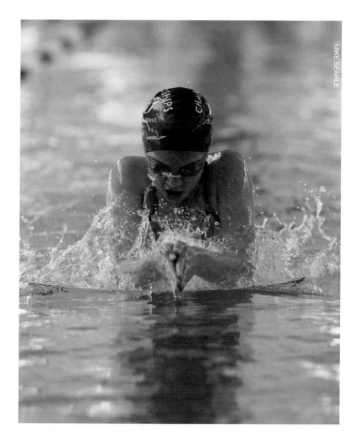

MIKE SEARLE

As a surfer, taking your heart rate up past the high end level of aerobic fitness and across to anaerobic training can be highly beneficial, as this would be very near maximal effort in running or swimming terms and is known as high anaerobic. You've probably got this high when the swell is cranking and the paddle out is rippy and hard work.

Understanding just what your body is put through will allow you to overcome these moments of exhaustion. Through heart rate monitoring during your training a higher level of fitness may well be achieved.

If you don't fancy using the HR system then you can try the "Perceived Rate of Exertion" chart. This is a very simple system and can be used by everybody at all levels of fitness.

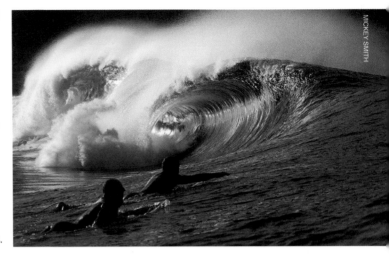

MICKEY SMITH

PERCEIVED RATE OF EXERTION CHART:

Activity	Scale	Heart Rate
At rest	1	Non exercise heart rates
Low level activity – sitting or walking	2	Non exercise heart rates
Light exertion such as a gentle jog	3	Non exercise heart rates
Normal walk	4	Non exercise heart rates
Brisk walking	5	Non exercise heart rates
Medium to fast paced walking	6	60% MHR low end aerobic
Breathing becomes more difficult	7	65%-75% MHR mid end aerobic
Breathing very heavily, talk just ok	8	80% MHR high end aerobic
Sweating, talk not possible	9	85%+ MHR anaerobic +
Max effort hard to maintain	10	90-100% MHR

A GUIDE TO COMPARE LEVEL OF TRAINING TO % MAX HEART RATE:

LEVEL OF TRAINING	% MAX HEART RATE
Low end aerobic training	60-70%
Mid end aerobic training	70-80%
High end aerobic training	85%+

LOW END AEROBIC TRAINING

low intensity would be around 60-70% of your max Heart Rate (HR)

MID END AEROBIC TRAINING

mid range intensity would bo around 70-80% of your max HR

HIGH END AEROBIC TRAINING

sub maximal high level intensity would be 85%+ of your max HR

SWIM TRAINING
PROGRAMMES

SWIMMING PROGRAMMES - BEGINNER

Each programme is broken up into 16 weeks, which cover 2 weeks training per phase, based on 2/3 sessions per week.

PHASE 1

Warm up
- Easy 8-10m minutes nonstop swimming

Main set
- 12x50m front crawl with 20 seconds rest in between each 50m (steady swimming)
- Then swim 12x25m as a sprint. Take max 60 seconds rest after each 25m
- Then swim 8-10 minutes nonstop as a swim down

PHASE 2

Warm up
- Easy 8-10 minutes nonstop swimming

Main set
- 14x50m front crawl with 20 seconds rest between each 50m (steady)
- Then swim 12x25m as a sprint. Take max 50 seconds rest after each 25m
- Then swim 8-10 minutes nonstop as a swim down

PHASE 3

Warm up
- Easy 8-10 minutes nonstop swimming

Main set
- 14x50m front crawl with 15 seconds rest between each 50m (steady)
- 12x25m as a sprint. Take max 40 seconds rest after each 50m.
- Swim 10-12 minutes nonstop as a swim down

PHASE 4

Warm up
- Swim 8-10 minutes nonstop swimming

Main set
- 16x50m front crawl with 15 seconds rest between each 50m (strong pace)
- 14x25m as a sprint take max 40 seconds rest after each 25m
- Swim 10-12 minutes nonstop as a swim down

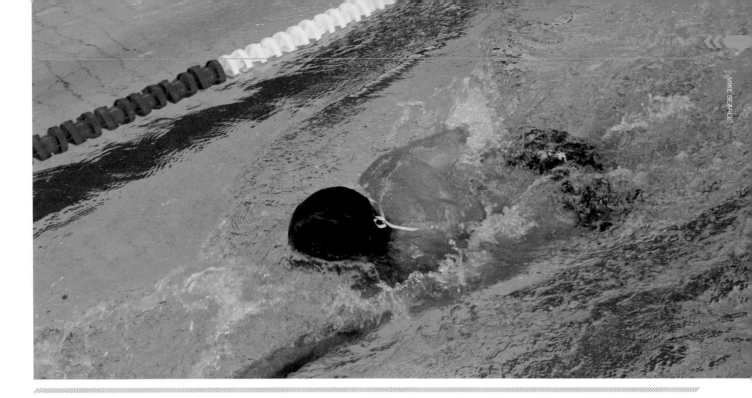

MIKE SEARLE

PHASE 5

Warm up
- Swim 8-10 minutes nonstop swimming

Main set
- 16x50m with 10 seconds rest between each 50m (strong pace). As your rest has now reduced to a minimal take an additional 60 seconds rest after you have reached half way (so after 8)
- 14x25m as a sprint, take max 30 seconds rest after each 25m
- Swim 10-12 minutes nonstop as a swim down

PHASE 6

Warm up
- Swim 10-12 minutes nonstop swimming

Main set
- 16x50m front crawl with 10 seconds rest between each 50m, and 60 seconds after 8
- 16x25m as a sprint, take max 30 seconds after each 25m
- Swim 12 minutes nonstop as a swim down

PHASE 7

Warm up
- Swim 10-12 minutes nonstop swimming

Main set
- 16x50m with 5 seconds rest between each 50m (strong pace) and 60 seconds rest after 8
- 16x25m as a sprint, take max 20-30 seconds after each 25m
- 12 minutes swim down

PHASE 8

Warm up
- Swim 10-12 minutes nonstop swimming

Main set
- 18x50m with 5 seconds rest between each 50m (strong pace), and 45 seconds after 10
- 18x25m as sprint, take max 20 seconds rest after each, and a further 60 seconds rest after 9
- 12 minutes swim down

SWIMMING PROGRAMMES - INTERMEDIATE

Again this programme is broken down into 8 two week phases, 16 weeks in total.

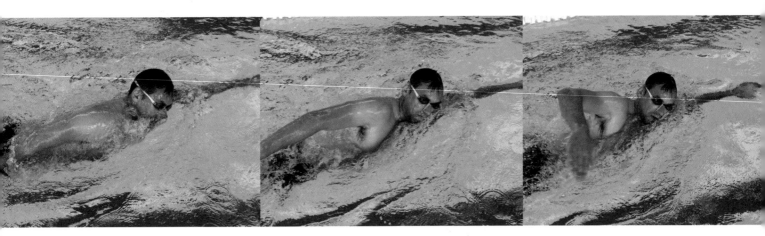

PHASE 1

Warm up
- 500m front crawl nonstop

Main set
- 10x75m front crawl with 20 seconds rest at a steady pace
- 8x25m front crawl with 30 seconds rest after each 25m as a sprint
- 5x75m front crawl with 20 seconds rest at a steady pace
- 8x25m front crawl with 30 seconds rest after each 25m as a sprint
- 400m swim down

PHASE 2

Warm up
- 500m front crawl nonstop

Main set
- 10x75m front crawl with 15 seconds rest at a steady pace
- 10x25m front crawl with 30 seconds rest after each 25m as a sprint
- 6x75m front crawl with 20 seconds rest at a steady pace
- 8x25m front crawl with 30 seconds rest as a sprint
- 1x50 front crawl sprint at MAX effort with 90 seconds rest
- 400m swim down

PHASE 3

Warm up
- 500m front crawl

Main set
- 10x75m front crawl with 10 seconds rest at a steady pace
- 10x25m front crawl with 20 seconds rest after each 25m as a sprint
- 6x75m front crawl with 20 seconds rest steady pace
- 8x25m front crawl with 15 seconds rest as a sprint
- 2x50m front crawl AS a sprint with 90 seconds rest
- 400m swim down

PHASE 4

Warm up
- 500m front crawl

Main set
- 12x75m front crawl with 10 seconds rest at a steady pace
- 10x25m front crawl with 20 seconds rest after each 25m as a sprint
- 6x75m front crawl with 20 seconds rest, steady pace
- 8x25m front crawl with 15 seconds rest as a sprint
- 3x50m front crawl as a sprint with 90 seconds rest
- 400m swim down

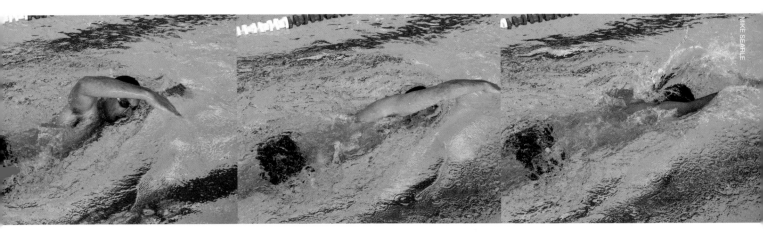

PHASE 5

Warm up
- 500m front crawl

Main set
- 12x75m front crawl with 10 seconds rest at a steady pace
- 10x25m front crawl with 20 seconds rest after each 25m as a sprint
- 6x75m front crawl with 20 seconds rest steady pace
- 8x25m front crawl with 15 seconds rest as a sprint
- 4x50m front crawl as a sprint with 90 seconds rest
- 400m swim down

PHASE 6

Warm up
- 500m front crawl

Main set
- 12x75m front crawl with 10 seconds rest at a steady pace
- 10x25m front crawl with 20 seconds rest after each 25m as a sprint
- 6x75m front crawl with 20 seconds rest steady pace
- 8x25m front crawl with 15 seconds rest as a sprint
- 5x50m front crawl as a sprint
- 400m swim down

PHASE 7

Warm up
- 500m front crawl

Main set
- 12x75m front crawl with 10 seconds rest at a steady pace
- 10x25m front crawl with 10 seconds rest after each 25m as a sprint
- 6x75m front crawl with 10 seconds rest steady pace
- 8x25m front crawl with 15 seconds rest as a sprint
- 5x50m front crawl as a sprint
- 400m swim down

PHASE 8

Warm up
- 500m front crawl

Main set
- 12x75m front crawl with 10 seconds rest at a steady pace
- 10x25m front crawl with 10 seconds rest after each 25m as a sprint
- 6x75m front crawl with 10 seconds rest steady pace
- 8x25m front crawl with 15 seconds rest as a sprint
- 6x50m front crawl as a sprint with 90 seconds rest
- 400m swim down

SWIMMING PROGRAMMES - ADVANCED

This advanced swimming programme is tough – it's likely that the swimmer/surfer will have at some point in their life been a competitive swimmer. Although the programme is still basic in comparison to an advanced programme for elite swimmers, it's still extremely well balanced for gains in surfing fitness.

PHASE 1

Warm up
- 600m front crawl

Main set
- 10x100m front crawl at a strong pace, 20 seconds rest
- 12x25m front crawl with 30 seconds rest as a sprint
- 5x100m front crawl with 20 seconds rest at a strong pace
- 12x25m front crawl with 20 seconds rest as a sprint
- 2 sets of 4x50m front crawl – take 60 seconds rest after each 50m as a sprint – then take an extra 2 minutes rest after each set of 4x50m
- 600m front crawl swim down

PHASE 2

Warm up
- 600m front crawl

Main set
- 10x100m front crawl at a strong pace, 15 seconds rest
- 12x25m front crawl with 30 seconds rest as a sprint
- 6x100m front crawl with 20 seconds rest at a strong pace
- 12x25m front crawl with 20 seconds rest as a sprint
- 2 sets of 4x50m front crawl – take 60 seconds rest after each 50m as a sprint – then take an extra 2 minutes rest after each set of 4x50m
- 600m front crawl swim down

PHASE 3

Warm up
- 600m front crawl

Main set
- 12x100m front crawl at a strong pace, 15 seconds rest
- 12x25m front crawl with 30 seconds rest as a sprint
- 6x100m front crawl with 20 seconds rest at a strong pace
- 12x25m front crawl with 20 seconds rest as a sprint
- 2 sets of 4x50m front crawl – take 60 seconds rest after each 50m as a sprint – then take an extra 2 minutes rest after each set of 4x50m
- 600m front crawl swim down

PHASE 4

Warm up
- 600m front crawl

Main set
- 14x100m front crawl at a strong pace, 10 seconds rest
- 12x25m front crawl with 30 seconds rest as a sprint
- 7x100m front crawl with 20 seconds rest at a strong pace
- 12x25m front crawl with 20 seconds rest as a sprint
- 2 sets of 4x50m front crawl – take 60 seconds rest after each 50m as a sprint – then take an extra 2 minutes rest after each set of 4x50m
- 600m front crawl swim down

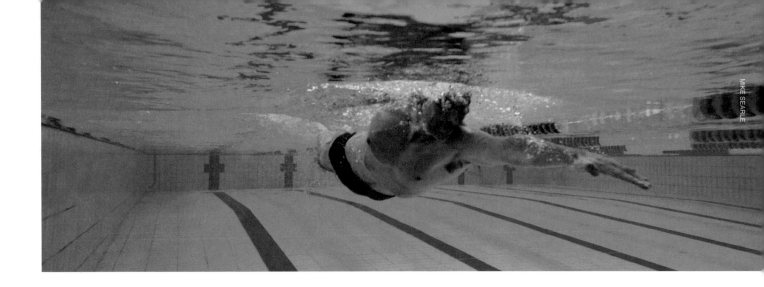

MIKE SEARLE

PHASE 5

Warm up
- 600m front crawl

Main set
- 14x100m front crawl at a strong pace, 10 seconds rest
- 12x25m front crawl with 20 seconds rest as a sprint
- 8x100m front crawl with 20 seconds rest at a strong pace
- 12x25m front crawl with 20 seconds rest as a sprint
- 2 sets of 4x50m front crawl – take 60 seconds rest after each 50m as a sprint – then take an extra 2 minutes rest after each set of 4x50m
- 600m front crawl swim down

PHASE 6

Warm up
- 600m front crawl

Main set
- 18x100m front crawl at a strong pace, 10 seconds rest
- 12x25m front crawl with 20 seconds rest as a sprint
- 8x100m front crawl with 20 seconds rest at a strong pace
- 12x25m front crawl with 20 seconds rest as a sprint
- 2 sets of 4x50m front crawl – take 60 seconds rest after each 50m as a sprint – then take an extra 2 minutes rest after each set of 4x50m
- 600m front crawl swim down

PHASE 7

Warm up
- 600m front crawl

Main set
- 20x100m front crawl at a strong pace, 10 seconds rest
- 14x25m front crawl with 20 seconds rest as a sprint
- 6x100m front crawl with 20 seconds rest at a strong pace – and last 25m of each 100m as a sprint
- 14x25m front crawl with 20 seconds rest as a sprint
- 2 sets of 4x50m front crawl – take 60 seconds rest after each 50m as a sprint – then take an extra 2 minutes rest after each set of 4x50m
- 600m front crawl swim down

PHASE 8

Warm up
- 600m front crawl

Main set
- 20x100m front crawl at a strong pace, 10 seconds rest
- 16x25m front crawl with 20 seconds rest as a sprint
- 6x100m front crawl with 20 seconds rest at a strong pace- and last 25m of each 100m as a sprint
- 16x25m front crawl with 20 seconds rest as a sprint
- 2 sets of 4x50m front crawl – take 60 seconds rest after each 50m as a sprint – then take an extra 2 minutes rest after each set of 4x50m
- 3x100m front crawl as a sprint with 90 seconds rest
- 600m front crawl swim down

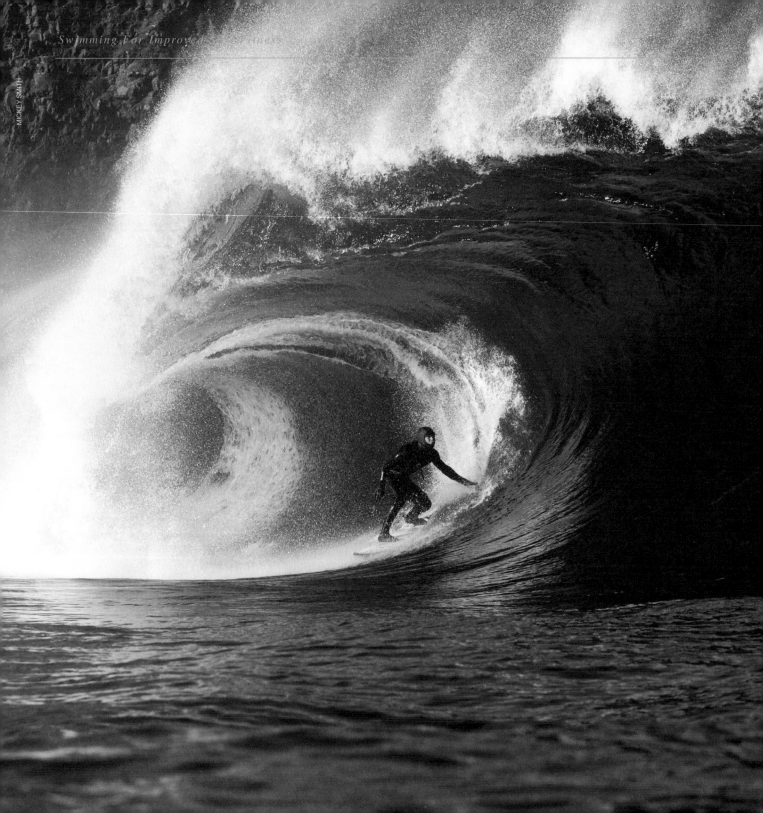

HYPOXIC SWIMMING TRAINING - ADVANCED

Breath holding or Hypoxic swimming training can be highly beneficial to a surfer. As most of us know a wipeout very often feels a lot longer than it is, and 10 seconds can feel like 40. Added to this, the fact that we are rolling around under water like a rag doll, especially in bigger waves, and things can feel pretty bad.

Basic swimming sets and holding your breath on a regular basis can really help. Try simple front crawl swimming, such as 12 x 25m holding your breath for each length, allowing as much rest as you need between lengths. When you're comfortable holding your breath, try swimming under water at the bottom of the pool, it is also a great way to build up your lung strength.

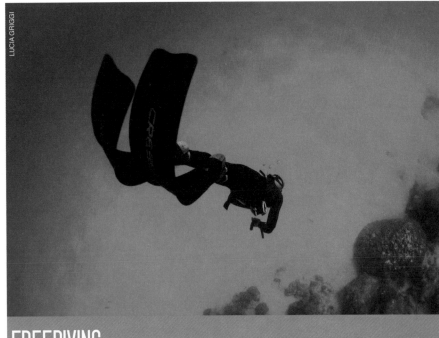

LUCIA GRIGGI

FREEDIVING

IF YOU GET THE CHANCE, TRY FREEDIVING TO BUILD UP YOUR LUNG STRENGTH AND FITNESS. PERFORMING BREATHING EXERCISES FOR FREE DIVING CAN HELP YOUR LUNGS BECOME CONDITIONED TO THE PHYSICAL DEMANDS REQUIRED FOR SURFING, ESPECIALLY BIG WAVE SURFING.

FLEXIBILITY& STRETCHING

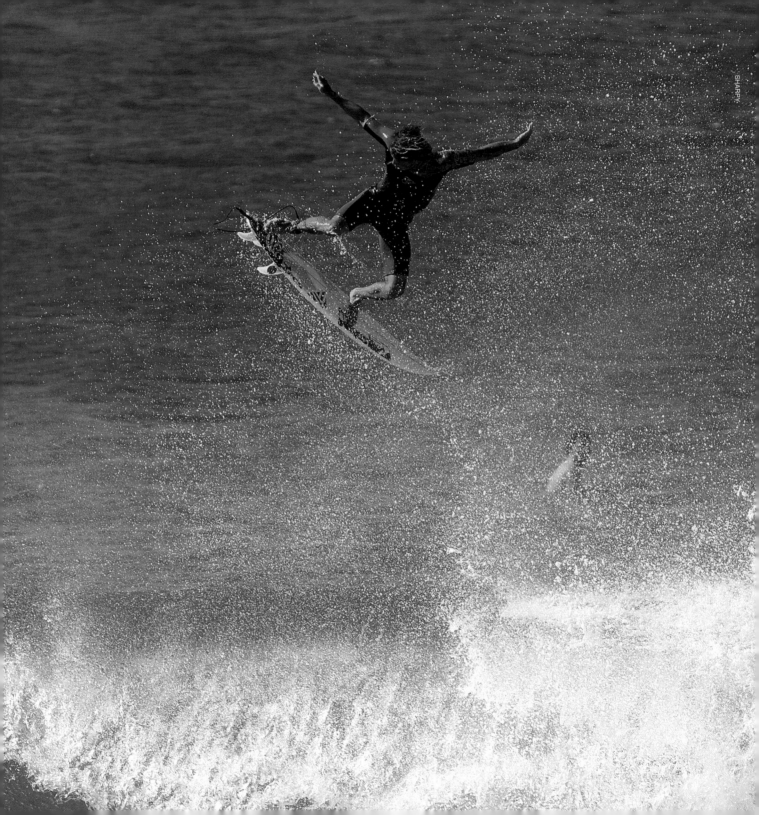

FLEXIBILITY FOR SURFING PERFORMANCE

A good flexibility programme can be the key to improved surfing performance. There is sometimes confusion, however, about just when is a good time to do a flexibility session stretch. Flexibility is a vital and often a neglected component of surfing performance, as it is a requisite for optimal musculoskeletal function.

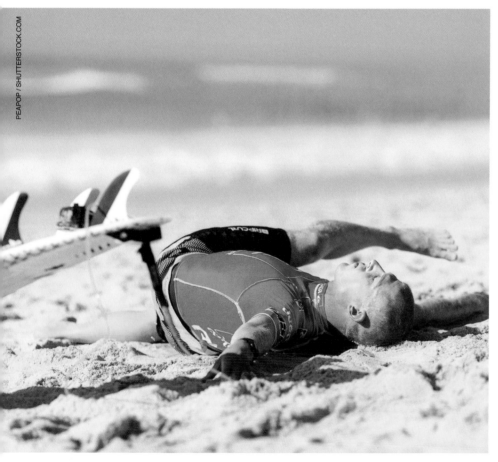

PEAPOP / SHUTTERSTOCK.COM

TYPES OF STRETCHING

There are various stretching techniques that can be employed to maintain, or indeed increase, flexibility for surfing. These are:

• STATIC

Slowly stretching a muscle to a point of mild discomfort/tension and maintaining this lengthened position for a set period; this can be up to 60 seconds.

Static stretching involves taking a joint through its range to a point where the soft tissue is comfortably stretched and then holding the position for a period of time. This may be done three ways: positional, active or passive. Static is the most well known stretching type and can be a safe and effective way of stretching after a surfing session, otherwise known as cool down stretching.

• DYNAMIC

Using controlled, rhythmical movement to take a joint through its normal range of movement (ROM).

Dynamic stretching is a controlled, rhythmic, repeated motion to the point of tension and return to full inner position. For example, from a seated position, extend one leg in front of you and draw the toes towards the knee (dorsal-flexion) until tension is felt, return to full toe point (plantar-flexion) and repeat 10 times. Each motion should take at least three seconds. By using controlled movements, this type of stretching also lubricates the joints by stimulating the production of synovial fluid. The combination of light activity and joint lubrication produces a combination of warm-up and stretching that is known as mobilisation, perfect for the many movements in surfing.

• PASSIVE

The term passive refers to the use of an external force, such as gravity, the use of another limb, or a partner to accomplish a stretch.

Passive static stretching is distinguished from assisted stretching by the absence (passive-static stretching) or presence (assisted stretching) of the sports massage

practitioner applying force. It will be further differentiated from positional or active static stretching by the addition of an external 'prop' or force. In passive-static stretching the athlete uses a prop to resist a force in order to extend or deepen a stretch. The prop may be as simple as using hand and arm strength to deepen a hamstring stretch, or a towel hooked over the heel to draw the leg into a deeper hamstring stretch. This is an effective way to deepen a positional static stretch, as the athlete is in control at all times. This type of flexibility training can be highly beneficial to surfers, however it's a type of flexibility training that is best left to the experienced professional.

• BALLISTIC

Rapid, bouncy, jerky movements performed at the end of the range of movement to facilitate stretching.

Ballistic stretching refers to a rapid, accelerative, repeated action beyond normal ROM with a slow return to the start position. It is the most controversial form of stretching as abnormal stretch reflexes can cause damage to the skeletal muscle unit or associated joint structures. It is necessary only in sport-specific instances where the declarative muscle is at risk of injury in explosive activities – for example, the hamstrings are at risk of injury

when they decelerate the knee as it approaches full extension during hurdling activities. Sprinters, hurdlers, martial artists and throwers are athletes who may need to incorporate ballistic stretching into their routines. This would follow other warm up and stretching activities to prepare the tissue, with this in mind this is not a good form of stretching for surfers.

• ACTIVE

In active static stretching one activates an isometric contraction (where force is exerted but muscle length does not change) at the full inner position of the joint – promoting the static stretch at extension of the antagonist muscle or group.

For example, fully contracting the hamstrings to full knee flexion will encourage a mechanical stretch of the quadriceps which will be enhanced by reciprocal inhibition. This type of stretching is useful for dancers and martial artists or others who need strength at extreme ranges of motion.

WHEN SHOULD I STRETCH?

There is often some confusion as to when it is best to stretch. As a basic rule, try not to over stretch before any exercise or hitting the water. Some light stretching can be done but it may be better to mobilise joints and ligaments and warm up muscles before any super long stretches take place.

PRE STRETCHES

The aim of the pre stretch is to help prepare the muscles for the forthcoming activity, thus reducing the risk of injury and enhancing performance. Pre stretches are traditionally performed after a warm up and target the muscle groups to be used in the exercise session. These are light stretches and do not form part of a developmental stretching programme.

These should be held at a point of mild tension for around 10 seconds.

MAINTENANCE STRETCHES

Maintenance stretches are performed post exercise or surf session and target the muscles used in that exercise or surf session. There function is to return the muscles to their pre-exercise length, thus maintaining the available ROM (range of movement), reducing soreness and aiding recovery.

Typically, they are held at a point of mild tension for approximately 10-20 seconds.

DEVELOPMENTAL STRETCHES

The aim of development stretches is to lengthen the muscle. It is generally performed at the end of a training session or on a separate occasion after a considerable warm up. Although there are various different ways in which developmental stretches can be performed essentially there are two phases:

1) A muscle is slowly stretched to a point of mild tension/discomfort and held in this position for around 6-10 seconds; This should be sufficient time for the stretch reflex to ease off.

2) At this point, the tension in the muscle should have reduced, allowing the muscle to be stretched a little further. These phases can be repeated several times, with the entire process lasting approximately 30 seconds.

Note: holding time for developmental stretches is typically 20-30 seconds plus. However a holding time of 30 seconds appears to be optimal with 15 seconds being less effective and 60 seconds being more effective.

GUIDELINES FOR STRETCHING

- It is important to remember that ALL stretches should be taught and performed in a slow and controlled manner, ensuring that participants are in a biomechanically sound position to facilitate the most effective stretch and reduce the risk of injury.
- Stretches aimed at developing flexibility should be held for about 30 seconds. Any developmental stretches undertaken particularly with young surfers should be done with care. If you are not sure of a particular stretching technique then you should consult a trained professional.
- For best results, stretching should be done on a regular basis. It's wise before undertaking flexibility routines to research in a constructive way so that a greater knowledge is gained of the many stretches available to the surfer or surf coach.
- It is very important to stretch to a point of mild tension/discomfort, and never stretch to the point of pain.
- Try to breathe normally while stretching and try to exhale when initiating a developmental stretch.
- Always aim for a well balanced stretching programme. During surfing sessions and movements many muscle groups are used, with the upper body, torso and pelvic areas being used widely.
- Always ensure a thorough warm up is performed prior to stretching.
- If you are with a small group of surfers (a surf club for example) then be aware of the whole group and monitor closely as poor stretching techniques can lead to injury.

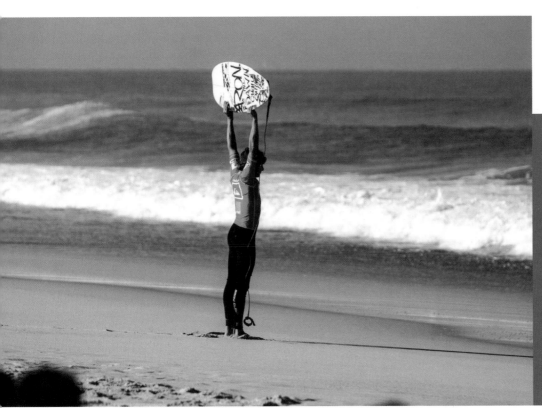

WHEN NOT TO STRETCH

- If there is or has recently been an injury to that muscle (in the last 3 days).
- If a joint is infected or inflamed.
- If a sharp pain is felt in the muscle or joint.
- If you are unsure of a particular stretch don't try it: seek advice!

SURFING INJURIES AND PREVENTION

The benefits of land based fitness training for surfing extends way past just being able to jump up on your board more effectively. The benefits are vast, one of which is injury prevention. Like in any sport, surfers will be at risk of an injury and at some point in a surfing life there's a good chance that it will happen!

Surfing is a very demanding sport, and the bigger the waves the more risk of injury there is. For any surfer an injury can be frustrating and with this in mind many surfers still feel there is no need to train on the land. However the benefits can mean much more than just catching a few extra waves.

// Look after your body

If you're lucky enough to get in the water on a regular basis then you're at risk of repetitious movements, such as those from non-stop paddling, which can take their toll on the body. Plus many surfers will not warm up or stretch after a surf and this is often why injuries creep in.

// Boost your core strength

Additional core strength can be a great benefit to any surfer, allowing additional strength to be gained in the back. During an average surf session the surfer will spend long periods of time with their lumbar spine (lower back) in constant extension (paddling). Then suddenly switch to reverse flexion (just before popping up) and this is where the lower back is often at risk from injury.

This is where a good land based training programme can be of benefit in the form of a good flexibility and stretching programme on a regular basis.

// Muscle strains

Muscle strain, pull or even a muscle tear implies damage to a muscle or its attaching tendons. You can put undue pressure on muscles during the course of normal daily activities, with sudden heavy lifting, during sports, or while performing work tasks.

Muscle damage can be in the form of tearing (part or all) of the muscle fibres and the tendons attached to the muscle. The tearing of the muscle can also damage small blood vessels, causing local bleeding (bruising) and pain (caused by irritation of the nerve endings in the area).

The amount of swelling or local bleeding into the muscle (from torn blood vessels) can best be managed early by applying ice packs and maintaining the strained muscle in a stretched position. Heat can be applied when the swelling has lessened. However, the early application of heat can increase swelling and pain.

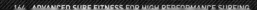

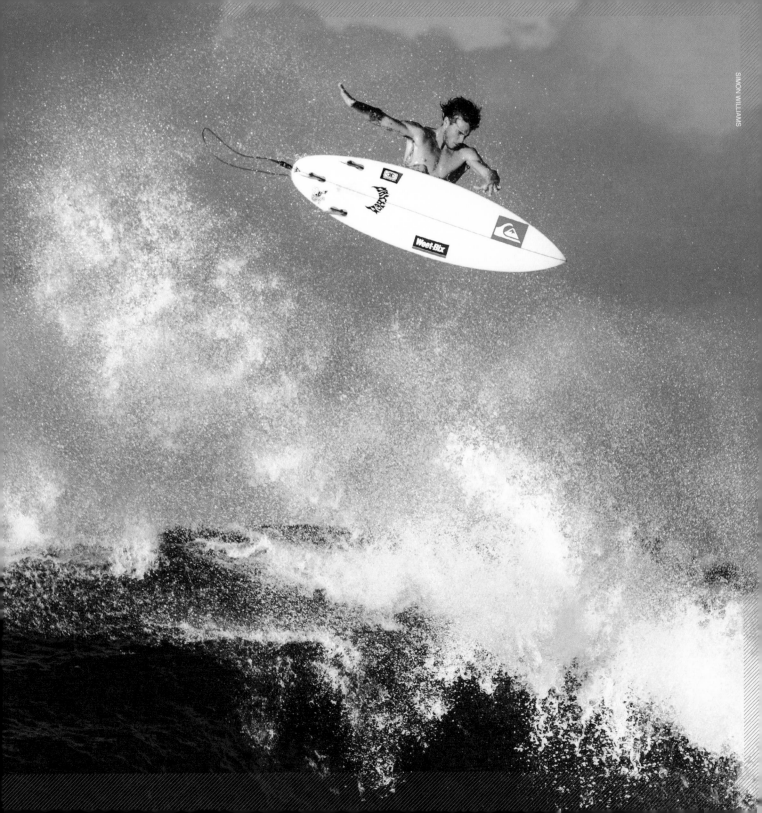

GETTING STARTED

WITH SOME FLEXIBILITY EXERCISES FOR IMPROVED SURFING PERFORMANCE

Many surfers (if they surf on a regular basis) have similar problem areas. This is often of course due to the fact that these areas are well used in surfing movements, like the hip flexors (pelvis area), adductors (between the legs) and shoulders. In many cases all that is needed is a good regular flexibility programme to solve their aches and pains

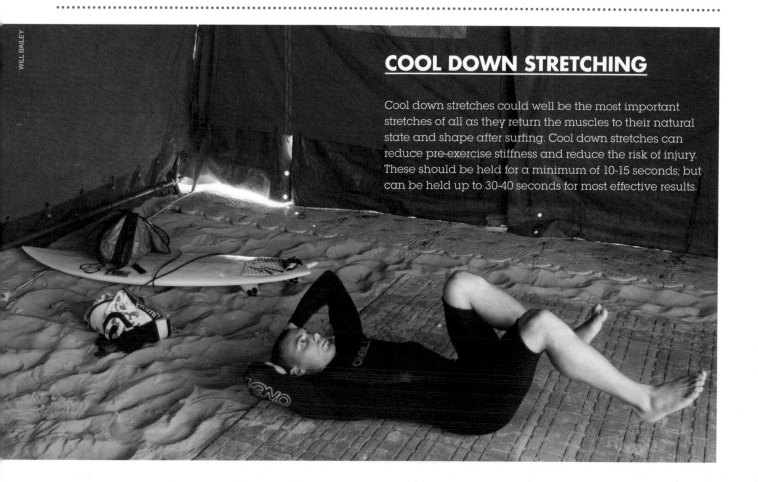

WILL BAILEY

COOL DOWN STRETCHING

Cool down stretches could well be the most important stretches of all as they return the muscles to their natural state and shape after surfing. Cool down stretches can reduce pre-exercise stiffness and reduce the risk of injury. These should be held for a minimum of 10-15 seconds; but can be held up to 30-40 seconds for most effective results.

POSSIBLE TARGET AREAS FOR SURFING FLEXIBILITY

SIT AND REACH STRETCH

Start by sitting on the floor with both legs out in front, then slowly reach forward to touch your toes – this will stretch the hamstrings and the spine. Aim for a smooth and controlled movement.

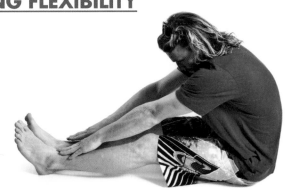

GLUTEAL STRETCH

The Gluteal muscles play a major role in surfing movements. They can often become tight, and a regular stretching programme can keep tightness and injury to a minimum.

Start the stretch by lying on the floor, with one leg extended, then try flexing the other leg. As you do pull it upwards and across towards your shoulder area. This stretch can also be done up against a wall but the effectiveness can be reduced.

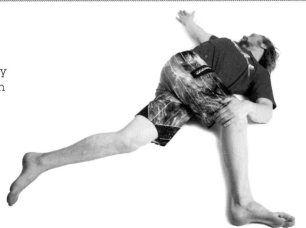

HIP ADDUCTOR STRETCH

The adductors are a group of 5 muscles that make up the musculature of the inner thigh. Their role is to bring the legs together, and during surfing movements on your board or during pop ups, these can become tight. Start by sitting on the floor with both legs extended then slowly flex your right leg and as you do so place your foot on your left thigh. Give a little support to your foot then press down slightly on the knee, as you do you should feel the stretch take place.

You may find that there is slightly more flexibility in one leg than the other; maintain good spinal alignment throughout the stretch.

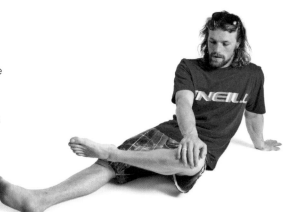

HAMSTRING STRETCH

Tight hamstrings can be painful and, as a surfer, taking care of this area is highly important.

Start the stretch by sitting with your right leg straight and your left leg bent. Then slowly reach forward with the right hand and grip the bottom of your foot, keeping the leg still and extended by lightly pressing on your knee.

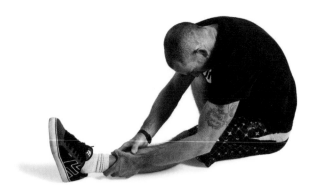

LOWER BACK STRETCH

The lower back can take a bit of a pounding due to the nature of paddling movements putting the back under pressure. With this in mind it would be wise to strengthen the back through training and adopt a good back flexibility programme.

Start by lying on the floor, draw your knees upwards towards your chest, grip hold of your knees and pull them into your chest and up towards your shoulders. Then allow your body to rock backwards and forwards which in turn will create a stretch in the spine.

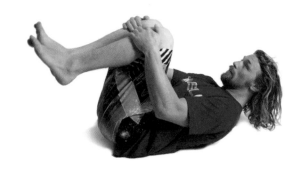

CAT STRETCH

A great stretch for your back, start the exercise on hands and knees, from here pull your tummy inwards, and slowly arch your back, hold for 20+ seconds then repeat.

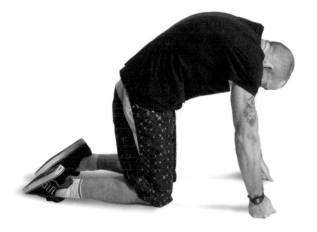

TRICEP STRETCH

Start with knees soft, pointing forward, feet about hip width apart. Take one arm up, keeping it close to the back of the head. From here slowly press lightly downwards on the elbow. Feel a light stretch on the back of the arm. Hold 20 seconds, then repeat on the other side.

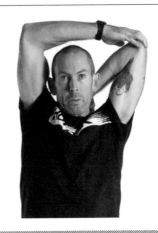

QUAD STRETCH

The quadriceps are the largest muscle group in the body and can be stretched in many ways. Try a simple stand on one leg with knees together. Slowly pull your foot upwards towards the buttocks and hold 20 seconds, then repeat.

If you're a little wobbly then hold a wall, or grab some support from a training partner.

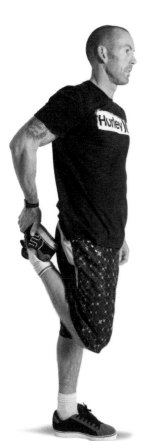

HIP FLEXOR HALF LUNGE STRETCH

Start by kneeling on your left leg with your right leg out in front of you. Aim for a good upright posture with good core stability, then press your right leg forwards. This should then help extend the left hip into a stretch.

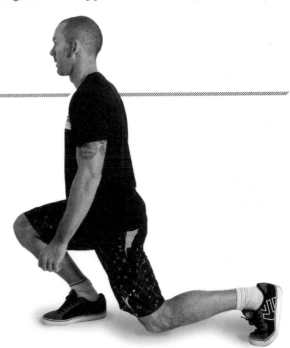

THE NECK STRETCH

If you're just about to hit the water a light 8-10 second neck stretch is important. The muscles around your shoulders will be used during paddle movements. It's important to mobilise and stretch your neck muscles as they offer support to this area. You can go for a longer stretch after your workout or surf.

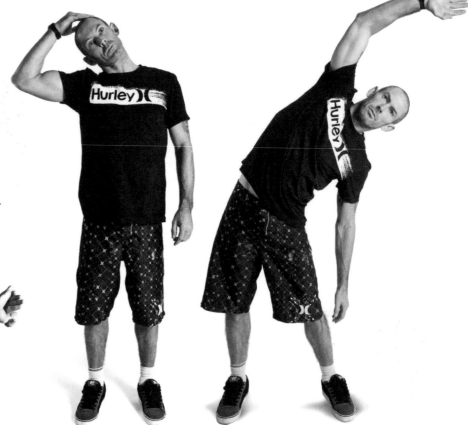

UPPER BACK STRETCH

This stretch can be done sitting or standing. Start by placing both hands out in front of you, then slowly push forwards. You will feel a stretch take place across your upper back. If you're standing keep feet pointing forwards, and if you're sitting just have your feet out in front of you,

LAT STRETCH

Another great stretch after a work out is the lat stretch. Great for the lats and spine. Start with soft knees, feet about hip width apart. Then slowly reach sidewards, hold for 20 seconds then repeat.

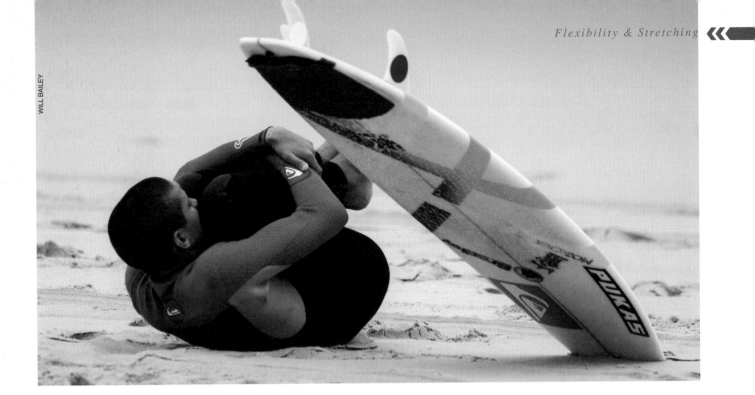

WILL BAILEY

Type of stretch	Duration	Muscles targeted
Hip Adductor stretch	30 seconds	Inside of the thigh including the groin
Glutei stretch	30 seconds	The bottom muscles
Hip flexor half lunge stretch	30 seconds	Found around the front area of the hips
Hamstring stretch	30 seconds	The back of your legs
Lower back stretch	30 seconds	Back, legs, buttock, and around the spine
Sit and reach stretch	30 seconds	Lower back and hamstrings
The Neck Stretch	30 seconds	Neck muscles: trapezius, scalenes levator scapulae
Upper back Stretch	30 seconds	Upper shoulder muscles and shoulder blades
Cat Stretch	30 seconds	Erector spinae and spine
Triceps stretch	30 seconds	Back of the arms
Lateral stretch	30 seconds	Lateral abdominal muscles and erector spinae
Quadriceps stretch	30 seconds	The muscle group at the front of each thigh

These are just a few example of good stretches after your surf. A well balanced flexibility programme after training and surfing will get the best results.

VISUALISATION TECHNIQUES FOR IMPROVING CONFIDENCE

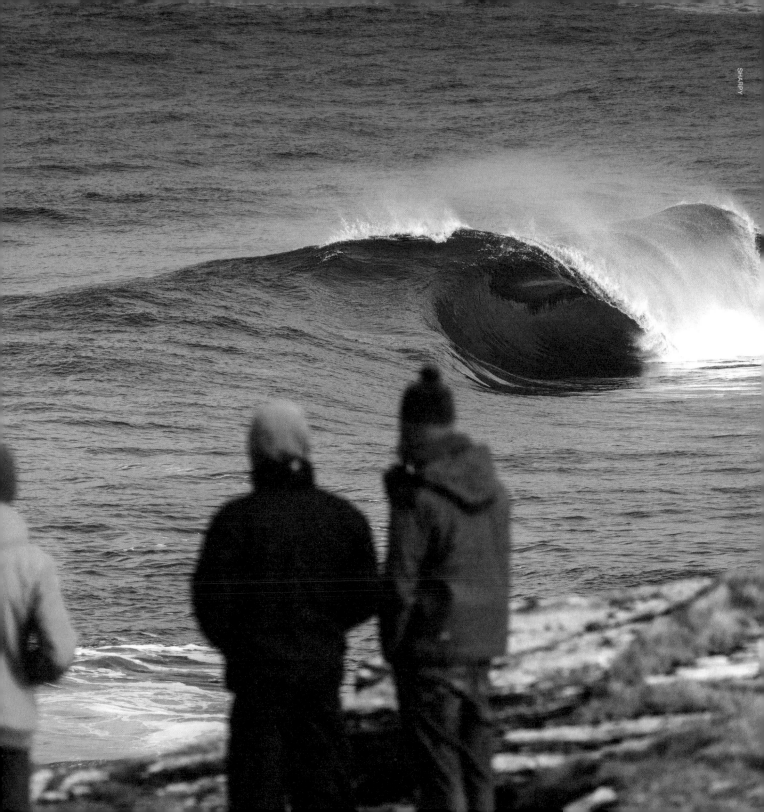

VISUALISATION TECHNIQUES
FOR SURFERS

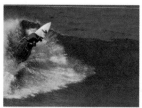
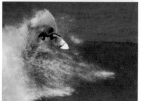
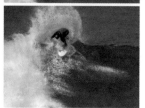
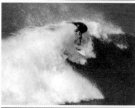
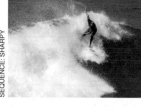

SEQUENCE: SHARPY

The skill of visualising sporting movements just before performance can take a bit of practice. However, once you've got over the basics, the benefits will truly boost your surfing. Many athletes across the world use visualisation techniques to boost their skills – and it's not just for pro surfers. In fact many surfers do it routinely without even realising it. Visualisation training can help sharpen the brain and create mental awareness before hitting the water.

The process is simple; you think about a move you want to do well, and then break it down in your mind over and over again. This then prepares the brain for the movements that will follow. This type of training can take place the day before a major comp, or just minutes before you paddle out. What is known for definite is that it really works in preparing the body for performance, and most top surfers will at some point use it.

If you're a competing surfer and you have an upcoming heat, find yourself a quiet corner way before your call up time, go over all that you want to achieve and picture what the surfing conditions are like that day, how your body will feel through that move and what possible scenarios might occur.

QUICK SUMMARY OF VISUALIZATION

- Keep your visualization drills simple.
- Try to make your images clear in your mind – just focus on the surfing move you want to improve.
- Do a prep of your mental work by watching the surfing move you are going to visualise. This will get your brain in gear and then reinforce your visualisation session.
- If you're about to visualize a surfing movement try taking it to the next level (focus on a more advanced version of the move), you may find yourself doing it out in the water without even thinking about it!

TRAIN INSANE OR
REMAIN THE SAME

SURF AND PREPARE TO WIN

Modern day performance surfing has now become much more than just jumping in the sea and trying to score points. Preparation takes place in so many areas now, from training in the gym to video analysis. Competition surfers are athletes, and prepping like a top athlete is the key to success.

#1 PREP FOR YOUR COMP DAY

- Give yourself a check list the night before. This will probably include top tips from your surf coach.
- Give yourself plenty of time to arrive at your competition.
- Check out your first heat time. Once you know your heat time make sure you plan that in to your warm up.
- Stay warm. Don't allow your core body temp to drop, this will affect performance.
- Stay hydrated right from the moment you wake up, keep a drink bottle to hand. Water will be fine, sports drinks are also fine, however try to drink water thoughout the morning. Dehydration affects the way you perform.
- Eat a decent breakfast. For sporting activity and competition, slow release carbohydrates are key. Cereals like porridge are a great way to start the day before competition.
- Once you know your heat time start preparing at least 20 minutes before.

#2 VISUALISE AND MOBILISE

- Warming up for your heat is key. Your mobility should last at least 10 minutes. Start from the top i.e. your head and move downwards, shoulders, arms, spine, hips, and ankles.
- Don't waste too much time stretching, you may wish to do a few short stretches but mobilising the key parts of your body for good surfing movements will be much more important. After your heat is the best time to stretch – this will allow your body to recover, and prepare for the next heat, if you have one.
- During your mobility session, start to seriously think about what your coach has advised you. For example the key areas of your surfing that need attention.
- Check the current surfing conditions. Start to visualise and think how best you will paddle out and where you will position yourself.
- Visualise a movement you may wish to implement for maximum points. Think about yourself doing the movement 8-10 times, and don't get distracted by anybody.
- Visualising before a sporting competition has been used by sportsmen and women for many years. Focus on your surfing movements before you do them and this will prepare your body.

#3 AFTER YOUR HEAT

- Any top athlete after their event will know the benefits of post exercise stretching, cooling down, and preparing the body with an 8-10 minute stretching routine.
- Preparing for your heat at a surfing comp in a serious and professional manner should only be part of any young surfer's regime.
- A healthy lifestyle directed around good and progressive surfing performance should be the main focus.
- Eat a healthy well balanced diet.
- Always stay well hydrated.
- Avoid junk foods.
- Build a solid base of surf fitness.

#4 KEY AREAS TO FOCUS ON FOR BOOSTING SURFING PERFORMANCE

- Balance training.
- Improve your core strength.
- Build a solid base of aerobic fitness.
- Build strength and endurance.
- Improve flexibility.
- Improve explosive power.
- Always use mobility whenever possible.

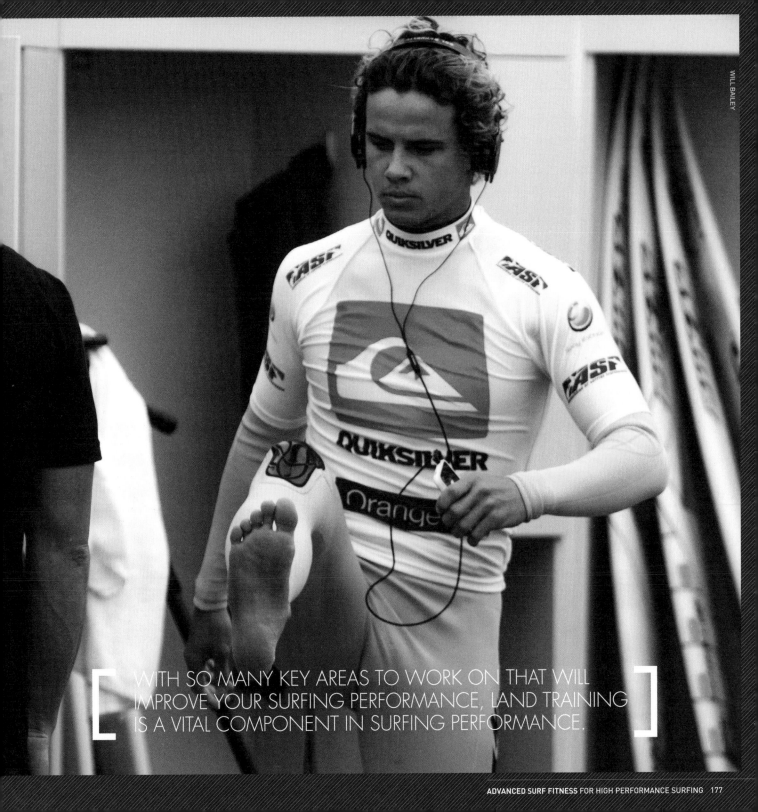

WILL BAILEY

[WITH SO MANY KEY AREAS TO WORK ON THAT WILL IMPROVE YOUR SURFING PERFORMANCE, LAND TRAINING IS A VITAL COMPONENT IN SURFING PERFORMANCE.]

"MY LIFESTYLE, MY TRAINING, MY OUTLOOK; EVERYTHING HAD SOMETHING TO DO WITH MY [WORLD TITLE] PERFORMANCE."

– MICK FANNING

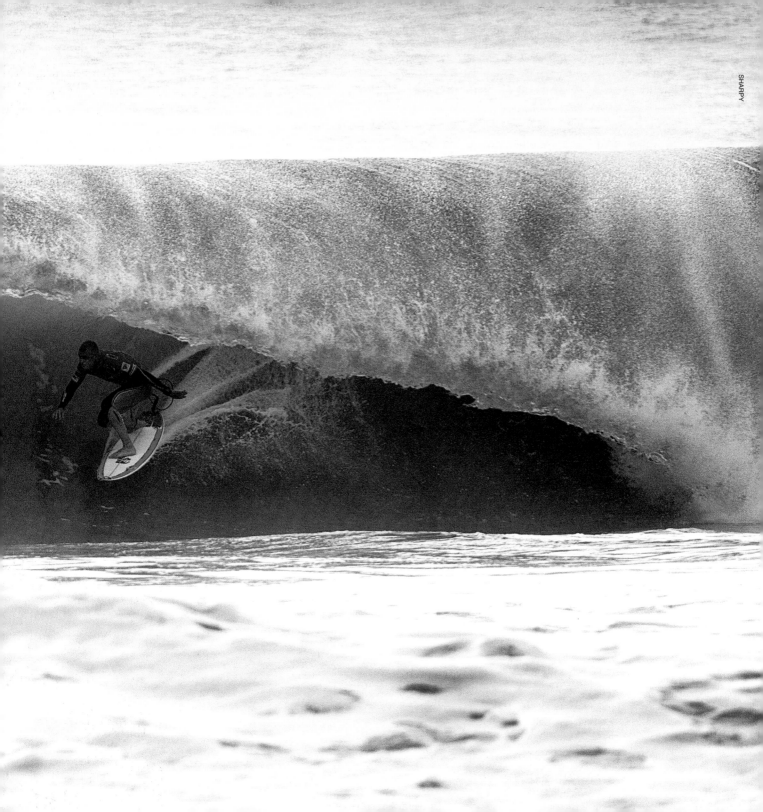

NUTRITION

A healthy balanced diet is crucial to your long term health and fitness. Good food choices will help give you fuel for training and help with recovery after your session.

If you're serious about a healthy surf fitness lifestyle then an organised approach to your nutrition is key. Bad eating habits will most definitely not fuel your surfing performance and fitness.

A varied and well balanced diet should provide you with adequate amounts of all the essential ingredients necessary for your training.

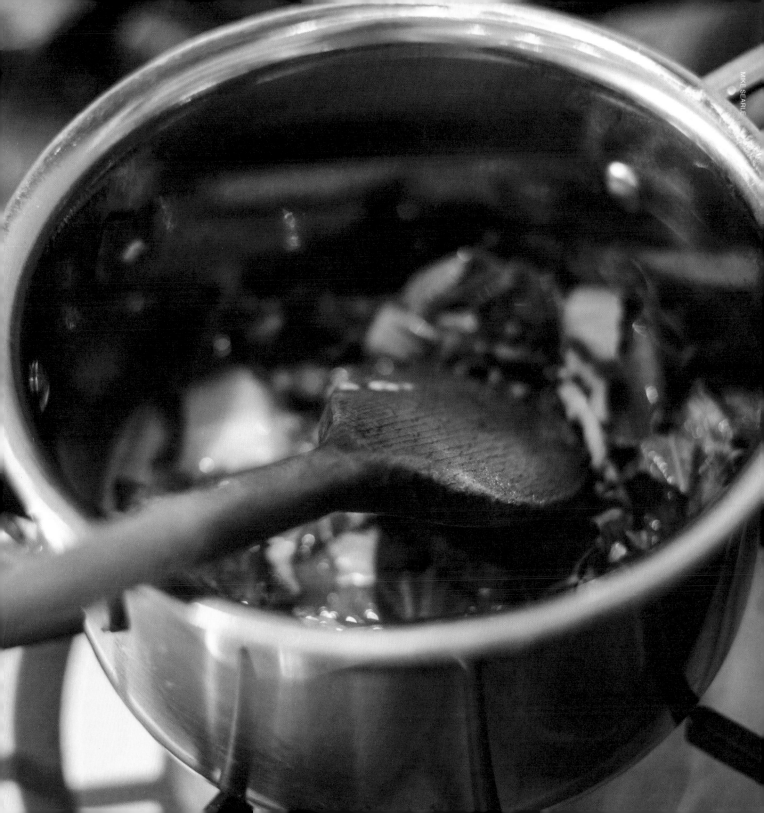

THE GOOD FOOD LIST

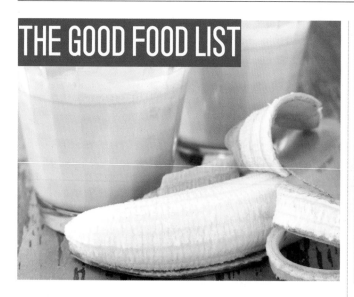

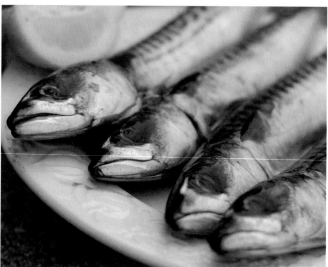

CARBOHYDRATES

Carbohydrates are the key ingredient for energy. During intensive activity the focus should be on carbs so that your energy tank is full and ready for take-off. They need to be regularly topped up as our stores of carbs are small. It's the most important energy fuel and crucial for sustaining training and recovery.

Good sources of carbohydrates are:

Sweet Potato
Rice
Cous cous
Boiled and new potatoes
Pumpkin
Baked beans
Wholegrain and rye bread
Muesli
Oatmeal
Whole-wheat pasta
Lentils

Brown rice
Berries
Dried apricots
Cashew nuts
Cereal

Fructose:
Banana (ripe)
Red Pepper
Pear
Apple

PROTEIN

Protein plays an important part in building and repairing muscle, and it is vital that a varied diet provides enough protein. A portion of protein is recommended within 30 minutes of exercise. Animal sources are richer than vegetable sources (so a larger quantity of non-animal sources needs to be consumed). Eggs are a good choice because they provide a good balance of protein and fat as are fish like salmon or haddock and low-fat dairy foods. Protein foods leave the stomach more slowly which means you stay fuller for longer.

Good sources of protein are:

Chicken and turkey
Pork
Fish
Soya beans
Tofu
Lentils
Kidney beans
Baked beans
Pistachio nuts

Eggs
Milk
Yoghurt
Cheese
Tuna
Pumpkin Seeds
Hummus
Almonds
Peanuts

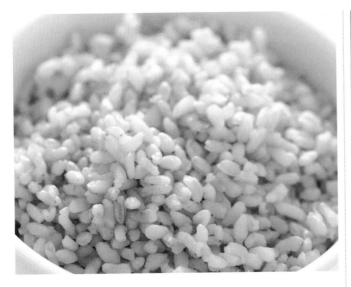

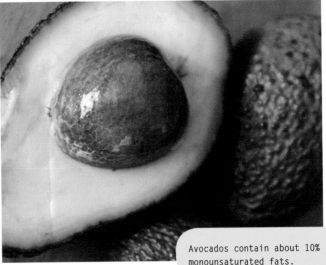

Avocados contain about 10% monounsaturated fats.

FIBRE

If you're surfing regularly and training hard you will need a good amount of fibre in your diet. High fibre foods are a great source of vitamins and minerals and also help prevent bowel problems. High fibre foods also fill you up for longer, can help keep weight down, and also help prevent heart disease by lowering LDL cholesterol.

Good sources of fibre:

Porridge	Jacket potato
Lentils	Wheat bran
Beans	Wholegrain cereals
Oats	Brown rice
Chickpeas	Fruit and vegetables
Walnuts	

Walnuts are a nutrient-dense food: 100 grams of walnuts contain 15.2 grams of protein, 65.2 grams of fat, and 6.7 grams of dietary fibre.

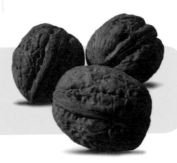

FATS

Fats play a highly important role in your surf fitness nutrition. Fats and·oils are made of fatty acids and serve as a rich source of energy for the body. Your body breaks down fats and uses them to store energy, insulate your body and transport vitamins through the bloodstream. It is true to say, however, that some fats are better than others!

• **Monounsaturated fats** are found mainly in vegetable oils like olive oil, and some peanut oils.

• **Polyunsaturated fats** are found mainly in vegetable oils like safflower, sunflower, corn, and flaxseed. They are also the main fats found in seafood.

• **Saturated fats** are mainly found in animal sources like meats and poultry, whole or reduced-fat milk and cheese.

• **Trans-fatty acids** can be formed when vegetable oils are processed into margarine or shortening. Sources of these trans fats include junk snack foods and baked goods made with partially hydrogenated vegetable oil or vegetable shortening.

ADOPT A GOOD FOOD PROGRAMME

Eat a wide variety of foods to ensure all your micronutrient requirements are met. You should get used to combining protein, fat and carbs in each meal or snack. So you need starchy carbs for breakfast and lunch to fuel activity, but for your evening meal the carbs are replaced by vegetables. You don't have to eat enormous meals to achieve this balance, in fact 4 or even 5 smaller meals a day can keep you trim, and as long as you eat the correct foods then this will help you maintain good energy levels into your surf competitions, training sessions and free surfs.

- Start each training session well hydrated. And after exercise aim to drink around 1.2 – 1.5 litres of fluid. Sports drinks provide both carbohydrate and fluid and are useful for intense exercise.
- Start a smart snacking programme. You will mostly likely see high sugar and high fat snacks advertised more than the healthy options, so plan out your snacks and give the unhealthy snacks a wide berth. Good choices are fresh fruit (especially bananas), natural cereal bars, nuts, raisins, oatcakes with hummus or cheese. These are also good pre-comp foods – in the build up to your heat snacks like this will keep you energy levels up. Start to refuel as soon as you can after exercise.
- Avoid sugary foods. Sugar is turned into glucose very easily which gives you an energy spike and leaves you feeling hungry sooner. If you crave sweet stuff try a few squares of dark chocolate and curb your temptations!
- If it's cold think about making flasks of hot liquid like hot blackcurrant or potato based soups for after your surf. It helps your body recover quicker.
- Eat green veg rather than starches with your evening meal. You're likely to be less active then so you won't need quick-release energy, but rather the slower release energy you'll get from these complex carbs.
- If it's late at night eating baked beans is better than not eating at all!

A SIMPLE DAILY GUIDELINE

If you're looking for a good vitamin and mineral balance that will aid your surf fitness training programme and allow you to perform well try these simple guide lines.

- 5 portions of fresh fruit and vegetables per day
- 2-3 portions dairy foods
- 3 portions protein
- 4-5 portions of breads/cereals

WHAT TRAINING IS BEST FOR STAYING 'SURF TRIM'?

A good mixture of exercises, although it's important to remember that steady aerobic training combined with some high intensity training is best.

During a high intensity workout or a heavy swell where you might paddle a lot most of your energy will come from glycogen – sugars stored in the liver and muscle fibres – however in general for the lower intensity surf or workout the energy will come from our fat stores.

RATES OF PERCEIVED EXERTION OR THE BORG SCALE

Although quite basic, this was developed by a psychologist named Gunnar Borg and uses a 10 point numerical scale to assess perceived exertion:

0	Basically nothing
0.5	Very ,very little output
1	Very Weak
2	Weak
3	Moderate
4	Somewhat hard
5	Hard
6	Harder
7	Very hard
8	Very very hard
9	Almost Sub Maximal
10	Very very Maximal

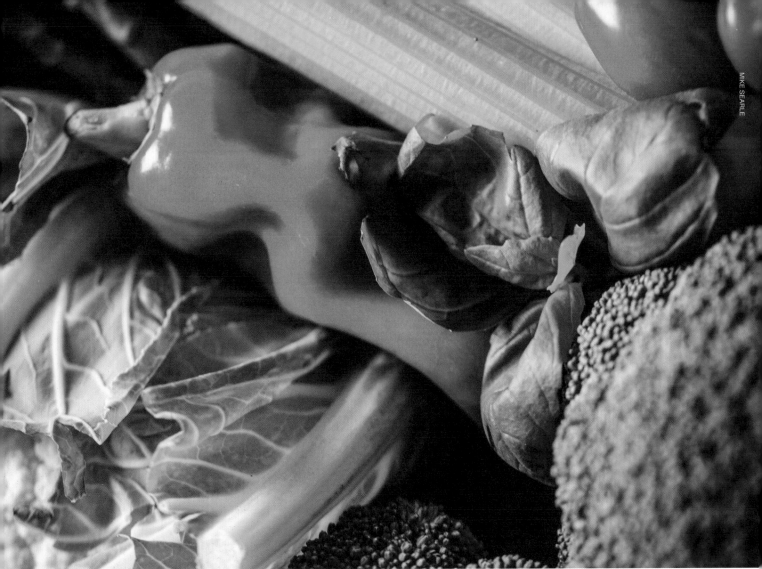

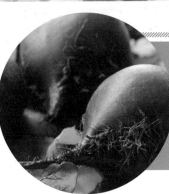

BEETROOT JUICE BOOSTS ENDURANCE

BEETROOT JUICE CAN BOOST STAMINA AND COULD HELP PEOPLE EXERCISE (AND SURF) FOR UP TO 16% LONGER. NITRATE CONTAINED IN THE VEGETABLE LEADS TO A REDUCTION IN OXYGEN UPTAKE - MAKING EXERCISE LESS TIRING. BEETROOT JUICE REDUCES VO2 LEVELS DURING MODERATE INTENSITY EXERCISE.

With an increasingly well-balanced diet you will see improved performance, and in addition to minerals and vitamins, there are also antioxidants which have their own benefits.

WHAT ARE ANTIOXIDANTS?

Antioxidants include Vitamins A, C, E and zinc, as well as enzymes that offer further support to our bodies, particularly when we are in training. Eating a variety of fruit and vegetables, which are good sources of antioxidants, will help support your surf fitness training programme.

HERBS

Herbs are found in many products. Natural herbs are best but herbs are also found in liquid extracts and teas. Fresh herbs from your garden can be a great side-line for supporting your surf fitness training programme.

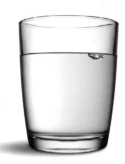

WATER

Water is vital to health as all body cells need water to function. If you do not take in enough fluids or if you lose fluids through vomiting or diarrhoea, you can become dehydrated and your surf fitness training will most definitely be effected.

During training hydration is highly important – having a glass of water every 15-20 minutes of training should keep you hydrated.

WHY DO WE STORE FAT?

Otherwise known as adipose tissue, fat is found all over the body. It acts as an insulator from the cold (but you will still need a 5mm in an English winter unless you're super tough or don't feel the cold). The body also stores fat around internal organs to help give them protection.

Fat metabolism and energy release
The fat tissue is made up mostly of lipid filled fat cells known as adiposities, which are stuck together with collagen fibres. These are energy rich and start to activate energy release once the glycogen starts to deplete. Once additional energy is required then the fats can be released from the tissue by a process known as lipolysis.

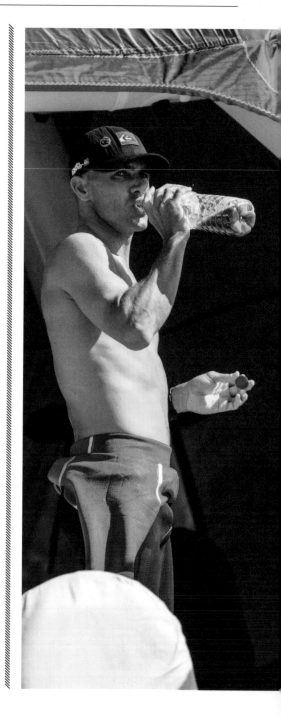

ARE YOU GETTING ENOUGH VITAMINS IN YOUR DIET?

Believe it or not our bodies only really need a small amount of vitamins and minerals to function well, keep illness away, and support brain function, the immune system, and the nervous system.

Here's a basic breakdown of a vitamin's function and where you can find it.

VITAMINS...

VITAMIN	FUNCTION	SOURCE
Vitamin A	Good eyes, skin, and healthy bones	Milk, butter, eggs, dark green veg, dark fruits
Beta carotene	Helps prevent infections	Fruits and vegetables
B1 Thiamine	Used in energy breakdown, healthy nerves	Meat, nuts, most whole grains
B2 Riboflavin	Healthy skin, supports vision	Dairy products, dark green veg, whole grains
B3 Niacin	Used in energy release	Meat, milk, eggs, meat fish, whole grains
Vitamin 12	Building blocks of new cells	Meat, milk, eggs, meat fish,
Folic acid	Helps form new cells	Liver, green veg, beans, nuts
Vitamin C	Antioxidants, helps fight infection	Citrus fruit, broccoli, tomatoes, melons, dark green veg
Vitamin D	Strong bones and teeth	Milk, eggs, liver
Vitamin E	Antioxidants , aids cell development	Vegetable oils, green veg
Vitamin K	Aids blood clotting	Green leafy veg, cabbage, liver

AND MINERALS...

MINERAL	FUNCTION	SOURCE
Calcium	Strong Bones, teeth, muscle contraction, blood and nerve function	Milk, green veg, salmon, shrimps, some fruit juice
Chloride	Good fluid balance	Salt, processed foods
Chromium	Aids energy release	Meat, wholegrain, veg oil
Fluoride	Formation of the bones and teeth	Water and toothpaste
Iodine	Helps the production of thyroid hormone	Iodised salt, and seafoods
Iron	Helps with the production of haemoglobin which carries oxygen round the body	Red meat, eggs, some breads, green veg, some dried fruit
Magnesium	Helps develop good bones and teeth	Meat, eggs, some breads, green veg, nuts
Sodium	Aids good fluid balance	Found in many foods
Sulphur	Part of protein, and thiamine	Protein rich foods
Zinc	Helps activate enzymes	Meat, poultry, fish

TRAINING PROGRAMMES AND PUTTING IT ALL TOGETHER

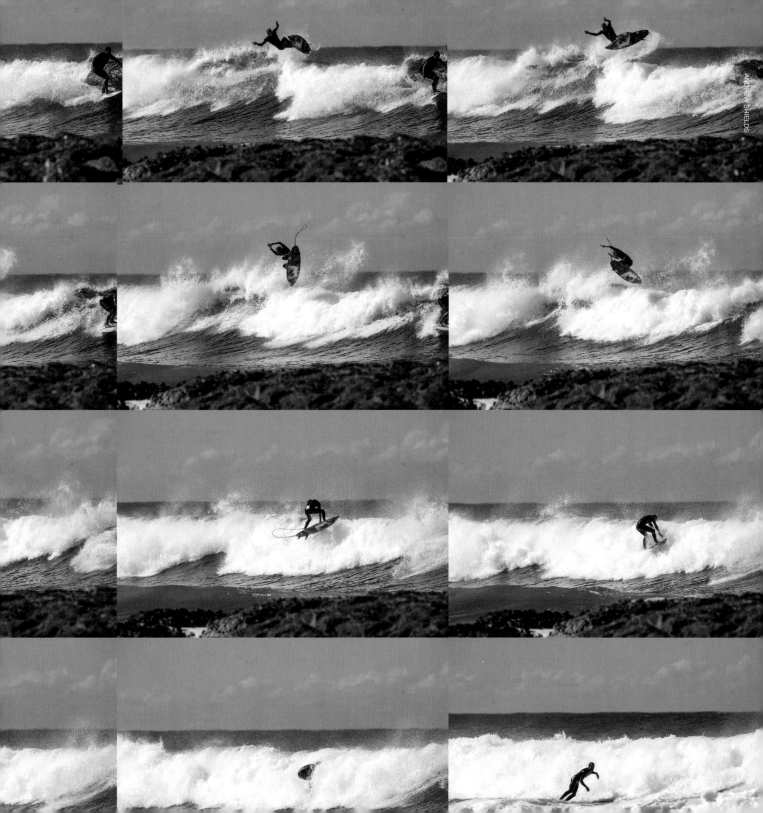

5 WEEK BASIC

A BASIC LEVEL OF FITNESS IS REQUIRED HERE. EASE INTO THIS PROGRAMME IF YOU'RE NEW TO FITNESS OR OUT OF PRACTICE.

KEY

+15   15 second rest between sets.
+20   20 second rest between sets.

SWIMMING

In the evenings on training days, try to aim for 60 minutes swimming. Follow the lay out of the swim training programme - page 153.

Follow this simple programme in total 6 sessions.

WEEK 1

MONDAY, WEDNESDAY AND FRIDAY

AM

- Warm up 8-10 minutes – starting with 3-4 minutes of mobility, then follow with 3-4 minutes of light aerobic activity.

Core set
- 6x30 seconds front plank +20
- 6x30 seconds side plank +20

Basic Plyometric set
- 5x8 basic upward jumps – with 30-45 rest after each 8 jumps

Core, and dynamic power set
- Indo Twists (or without Indo Board) 12x20 seconds of the exercise then 60 seconds rest

Strength and Endurance Set
- 6x8 press ups +20
- Light weight - 4x5 reps front raises +20
- Light weight - 4x5 reps side raises +20
- Light weight - 4x5 reps shoulder press +20
- Light weight - 4x5 reps triceps drop +20
- Light weight - 4x5 reps basic squats +20
- Light weight - 4x5 reps reverse flyes +20
- Walking lunges – with light weight, 4x5 reps +20

Cool down
15 minutes, light aerobic jog, followed by stretching

- Adductor stretch 4x20 +30
- Gluteal stretch 4x20 +30
- Hamstring stretch 4x20 +30

PM
- **Swimming** 30 minutes.

WEEK 2

MONDAY, WEDNESDAY AND FRIDAY

AM

- Warm up 8-10 minutes – starting with 3-4 minutes of mobility, then follow with 3-4 minutes of light aerobic activity.

Core set
- 6x30 seconds front plank +20
- 6x30 seconds side plank +20

Basic Plyometric set
- 5x8 basic upward jumps – with 30-45 rest after each 8 jumps

Core, and dynamic power set
- Indo Twists (or without Indo Board) 12x20 seconds of the exercise then 60 seconds rest

Strength and Endurance Set
- 6x8 press ups +20
- Light weight - 4x5 reps front raises +20
- Light weight - 4x5 reps side raises +20
- Light weight - 4x5 reps shoulder press +20
- Light weight - 4x5 reps triceps drop +20
- Light weight - 4x5 reps basic squats +20
- Light weight - 4x5 reps reverse flyes +20
- Walking lunges – with light weight, 4x5 reps +20

Cool down
15 minutes, light aerobic jog, followed by stretching

- Adductor stretch 4x20 +30
- Gluteal stretch 4x20 +30
- Hamstring stretch 4x20 +30

PM
- **Swimming** 30 minutes.

WEEK 3
MONDAY, WEDNESDAY AND FRIDAY

AM

- Warm up 8-10 minutes – starting with 3-4 minutes of mobility, then follow with 3-4 minutes of light aerobic activity.

Core set
- 6x30 seconds front plank +20
- 6x30 seconds side plank +20

Basic Plyometric set
- 5x8 basic upward jumps – with 30-45 rest after each 8 jumps

Core, and dynamic power set
- Indo Twists (or without Indo Board) 12x20 seconds of the exercise then 60 seconds rest

Strength and Endurance Set
- 6x8 press ups +20
- Light weight - 4x5 reps front raises +20
- Light weight - 4x5 reps side raises +20
- Light weight - 4x5 reps shoulder press +20
- Light weight - 4x5 reps triceps drop +20
- Light weight - 4x5 reps basic squats +20
- Light weight - 4x5 reps reverse flyes +20
- Walking lunges – with light weight, 4x5 reps +20

Cool down
15 minutes, light aerobic jog, followed by stretching

- Adductor stretch 4x20 +30
- Gluteal stretch 4x20 +30
- Hamstring stretch 4x20 +30

PM
- **Swimming** 30 minutes.

WEEK 4
MONDAY, WEDNESDAY AND FRIDAY

AM

- Warm up 8-10 minutes – starting with 3-4 minutes of mobility, then follow with 3-4 minutes of light aerobic activity.

Core set
- 6x30 seconds front plank +20
- 6x30 seconds side plank +20

Basic Plyometric set
- 5x8 basic upward jumps – with 30-45 rest after each 8 jumps

Core, and dynamic power set
- Indo Twists (or without Indo Board) 12x20 seconds of the exercise then 60 seconds rest

Strength and Endurance Set
- 6x8 press ups +20
- Light weight - 4x5 reps front raises +20
- Light weight - 4x5 reps side raises +20
- Light weight - 4x5 reps shoulder press +20
- Light weight - 4x5 reps triceps drop +20
- Light weight - 4x5 reps basic squats +20
- Light weight - 4x5 reps reverse flyes +20
- Walking lunges – with light weight, 4x5 reps +20

Cool down
15 minutes, light aerobic jog, followed by stretching

- Adductor stretch 4x20 +30
- Gluteal stretch 4x20 +30
- Hamstring stretch 4x20 +30

PM
- **Swimming** 30 minutes.

WEEK 5
MONDAY, WEDNESDAY AND FRIDAY

AM

- Warm up 8-10 minutes – starting with 3-4 minutes of mobility, then follow with 3-4 minutes of light aerobic activity.

Core set
- 6x30 seconds front plank +20
- 6x30 seconds side plank +20

Basic Plyometric set
- 5x8 basic upward jumps – with 30-45 rest after each 8 jumps

Core, and dynamic power set
- Indo Twists (or without Indo Board) 12x20 seconds of the exercise then 60 seconds rest

Strength and Endurance Set
- 6x8 press ups +20
- Light weight - 4x5 reps front raises +20
- Light weight - 4x5 reps side raises +20
- Light weight - 4x5 reps shoulder press +20
- Light weight - 4x5 reps triceps drop +20
- Light weight - 4x5 reps basic squats +20
- Light weight - 4x5 reps reverse flyes +20
- Walking lunges – with light weight, 4x5 reps +20

Cool down
15 minutes, light aerobic jog, followed by stretching

- Adductor stretch 4x20 +30
- Gluteal stretch 4x20 +30
- Hamstring stretch 4x20 +30

PM
- **Swimming** 30 minutes.

5 WEEK INTERMEDIATE

IT'S TIME TO TAKE THINGS UP A LEVEL. SO ONCE YOU'VE GIVEN YOURSELF A GOOD FOUR WEEK BASE, GO THE EXTRA MILE AND THIS WILL IMPROVE YOUR FITNESS FURTHER.

KEY

+15   15 second rest between sets.

+20   20 second rest between sets.

SWIMMING

In the evenings on training days, try to aim for 60 minutes swimming. Follow the lay out of the swim training programme - page 153.

Follow this simple programme in total 6 sessions.

WEEK 1

MONDAY, WEDNESDAY AND FRIDAY

AM

- Warm up 8-10 minutes – starting with 3-4 minutes of mobility, then follow with 3-4 minutes of light aerobic activity.

Core set
- 6x60 seconds front plank +20
- 6x30 seconds side plank +20

Basic Plyometric set
- 6x8 Double leg jumps in a row +20
- Light 10 minute jog
- 12x8 basic upward jumps – with 30-45 rest after each 8 jumps

Core, and dynamic power set
- Indo Twists (or without Indo Board) 14x 30 seconds of the exercise then 60 seconds rest

Strength and Endurance Set
- 6x12press ups +20 + 1 set as many as possible
- Light weight - 4x8 reps front raises +20
- Light weight - 4x8 reps side raises +20
- Light weight - 4x8 reps shoulder press +20
- Light weight - 4x8 reps triceps drop +20
- Light weight - 4x8 reps basic squats +20
- Light weight - 4x8 reps reverse flyes +20
- Walking lunges – with light weight, 4x8 reps +20

Cool down
15 minutes light aerobic jog, followed by stretching
- Adductor stretch 4x20 +30
- Gluteal stretch 4x20 +30
- Hamstring stretch 4x20 +30

PM
- **Swimming** 30 minutes.

WEEK 2

MONDAY, WEDNESDAY AND FRIDAY

AM

- Warm up 8-10 minutes – starting with 3-4 minutes of mobility, then follow with 3-4 minutes of light aerobic activity.

Core set
- 6x60 seconds front plank +20 + one set as long as possible
- 6x30 seconds side plank +20

Basic Plyometric set
- 6x10 Double leg jumps in a row +20 seconds rest
- Light 10 minute jog
- 12x8 basic upward jumps – with 30-45 rest after each 8 jumps

Core, and dynamic power set
- Indo Twists (or without Indo Board) 12x30 seconds of the exercise then 60 seconds rest

Strength and Endurance Set
- 6x10 press ups +20 + 0ne set as many as posible
- Light weight - 4x8 reps front raises +20
- Light weight - 4x8 reps side raises +20
- Light weight - 4x12 reps shoulder press +20
- Light weight - 4x12 reps triceps drop +20
- Light weight - 4x12 reps basic squats +20
- Light weight - 4x12 reps reverse flyes +20
- Walking lunges – with light weight, 4x10 reps +20

Cool down
15 minutes light aerobic jog, followed by stretching
- Adductor stretch 4x20 +30
- Gluteal stretch 4x20 -+30
- Hamstring stretch 4x20 +30

PM
- **Swimming** 30 minutes.

WEEK 3
MONDAY, WEDNESDAY AND FRIDAY

AM

- Warm up 8-10 minutes – starting with 3-4 minutes of mobility, then follow with 3-4 minutes of light aerobic activity.

Core set
- 6x90 seconds front plank +20 + one set as long as possible
- 6x40 seconds side plank +20

Basic Plyometric set
- 8x10 Double leg jumps in a row +20
- Light 10 minute jog
- 12x10 basic upward jumps – with 30-45 rest after each 10 jumps

Core, and dynamic power set
- Indo Twists (or without Indo Board) 12x30 seconds of the exercise then 60 seconds rest

Strength and Endurance Set
- 8x10 press ups +20 + 1 set as many as posible
- Light weight - 4x8 reps front raises +20
- Light weight - 4x8 reps side raises +20
- Light weight - 4x12 reps shoulder press +20
- Light weight - 4x12 reps triceps drop +20
- Light weight - 4x12 reps basic squats +20
- Light weight - 4x12 reps reverse flyes +20
- Walking lunges – with light weight, 4x10 reps +20

Cool down
15 minutes light aerobic jog, followed by stretching
- Adductor stretch 4x20 +30
- Gluteal stretch 4x20 +30
- Hamstring stretch 4x20 +30

PM
- **Swimming** 40 minutes.

WEEK 4
MONDAY, WEDNESDAY AND FRIDAY

AM

- Warm up 8-10 minutes – starting with 3-4 minutes of mobility, then follow with 3-4 minutes of light aerobic activity.

Core set
- 8x90 seconds front plank +20 + one set as long as possible
- 6x40 seconds side plank +20

Basic Plyometric set
- 10x10 Double leg jumps in a row +20
- Light 10 minute jog
- 12x10 basic upward jumps – with 30-45 rest after each 12 jumps

Core, and dynamic power set
- Indo Twists (or without Indo Board) 12x30 seconds of the exercise then 60 seconds rest

Strength and Endurance Set
- 8x10 press ups +20
- Light weight - 5x8 reps front raises +20
- Light weight - 5x8 reps side raises +20
- Light weight - 5x12 reps shoulder press +20
- Light weight - 5x12 reps triceps drop +20
- Light weight - 5x12 reps basic squats +20
- Light weight - 5x12 reps reverse flyes +20
- Walking lunges – with light weight, 5x10 reps +20

Cool down
15 minutes light aerobic jog, followed by stretching
- Adductor stretch 4x20 +30
- Gluteal stretch 4x20 -+30
- Hamstring stretch 4x20 +30

PM
- **Swimming** 40 minutes.

WEEK 5
MONDAY, WEDNESDAY AND FRIDAY

AM

- Warm up 8-10 minutes – starting with 3-4 minutes of mobility, then follow with 3-4 minutes of light aerobic activity.

Core set
- 6x90 seconds front plank +20 + one set as long as possible
- 6x40 seconds side plank +20

Basic Plyometric set
- 16x10 Double leg jumps in a row +20
- Light 10 minute jog
- 12x12 basic upward jumps – with 30-45 rest after each 8 jumps

Core, and dynamic power set
- Indo Twists (or without Indo Board) 12x30 seconds of the exercise then 60 seconds rest

Strength and Endurance Set
- 8x10 press ups + 20 seconds rest
- Light weight - 5x12reps front raises +20
- Light weight - 5x12 reps side raises +20
- Light weight - 5x12 reps shoulder press +20
- Light weight - 5x12 reps triceps drop +20
- Light weight - 5x12 reps basic squats +20
- Light weight - 5x12 reps reverse flyes +20
- Walking lunges – with light weight, 6x10 reps +20

Cool down
15 minutes light aerobic jog, followed by stretching
- Adductor stretch 4x20 +30
- Gluteal stretch 4x20 +30
- Hamstring stretch 4x20 +30

PM
- **Swimming** 40 minutes.

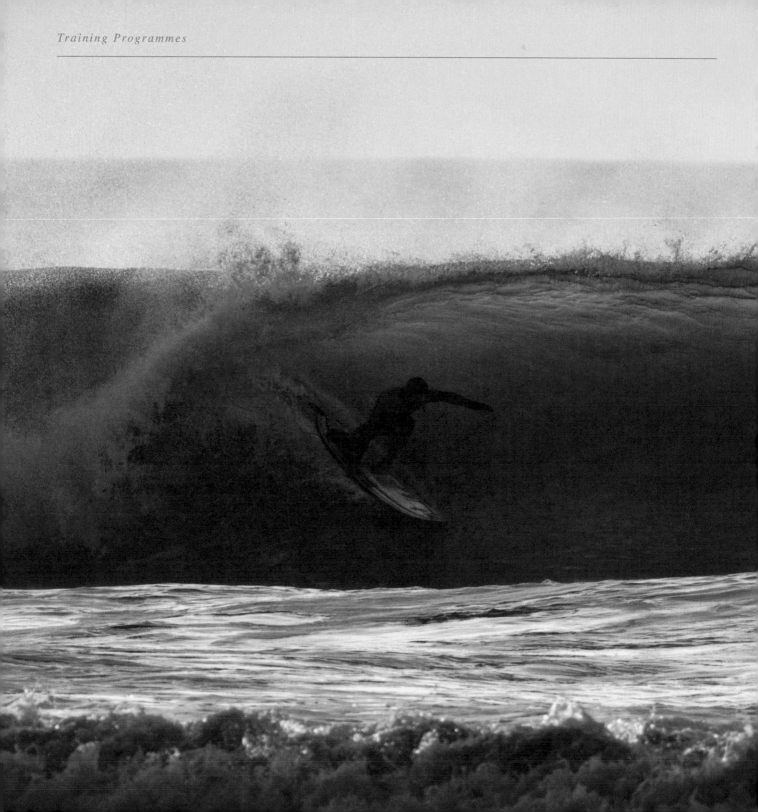

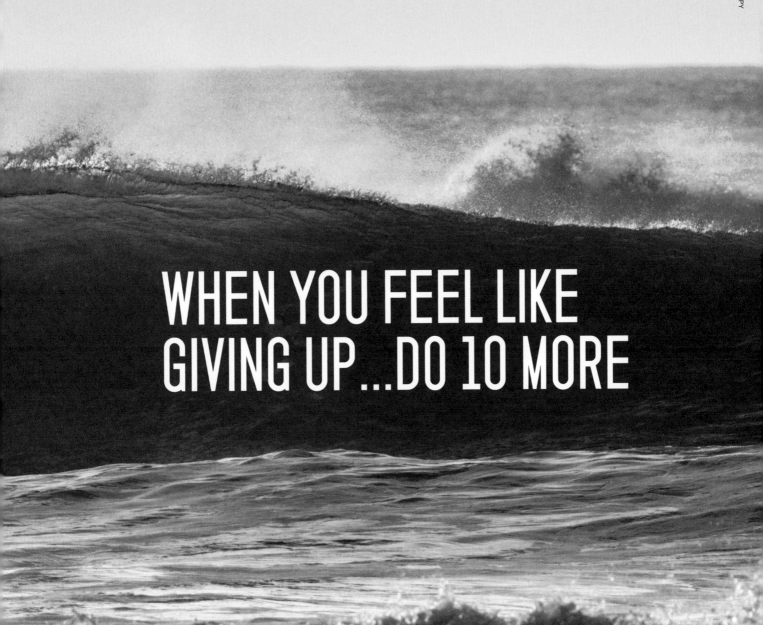

WHEN YOU FEEL LIKE GIVING UP...DO 10 MORE

16 WEEK ADVANCED

NOW YOU'RE GETTING MUCH FITTER YOU CAN REALLY STEP IT UP! WORKING HARD ON LONGER LENGTHS OF TRAINING, WITH GREATER INTENSITY WILL REAP FAR GREATER IMPROVEMENTS IN YOUR SURFING!

KEY
+15   15 second rest between sets.
+20   20 second rest between sets.

SWIMMING
In the evenings on training days, try to aim for 60 minutes swimming. Follow the lay out of the swim training programme - page 153.

Follow this simple programme in total 6 sessions.

WEEK 1
MONDAY, WEDNESDAY AND FRIDAY

AM
- Warm up 8-10 minutes – starting with 3-4 minutes of mobility, then follow with 3-4 minutes of light aerobic activity.

Core set
- 6x90 seconds front plank +20
- 6x30 seconds side plank +20

Basic Plyometric set
- 8x8 double leg jumps in a row with weight +20
- 12x8 basic upward jumps – with 30 rest after each 8 jumps.

Core, and dynamic power set
- Indo Twists (or without Indo Board) 12x30 seconds of the exercise then 60 seconds rest.

Strength and Endurance Set
- 6x15 press ups + 20 seconds rest
- Light weight - 4x12 reps front raises +20
- Light weight - 4x12 reps side raises +20
- Light weight - 4x12 reps shoulder press +20
- Light weight - 4x12 reps triceps drop +20
- Light weight - 4x12 reps basic squats +20
- Light weight - 4x12 reps reverse flyes +20
- Walking lunges - with light weight, 4x12 reps +20

Cool down
15 minutes light aerobic jog, followed by stretching
- Adductor stretch 4 x 20 +30
- Gluteal stretch 4x20 +30
- Hamstring stretch 4x20 +30

PM
- **Swimming** 60 minutes.

WEEK 2
MONDAY, WEDNESDAY AND FRIDAY

AM
- Warm up 8-10 minutes – starting with 3-4 minutes of mobility, then follow with 3-4 minutes of light aerobic activity.

Core set
- 10x90 seconds front plank +20
- 10x30 seconds side plank +20

Basic Plyometric set
- 6x 8 Double leg jumps in a row +20
- 6x8 spin and squat+20 no weight
- Light 10 minute jog
- 12x10 basic upward jumps - with 30-45 rest after each 8 jumps (use light weight).

Core, and dynamic power set
- Indo Twists (or without Indo Board) 14x30 seconds of the exercise then 60 seconds rest.
- 6x6 Spin and stick on BOSU +20

Strength and Endurance Set
- 6x12 press ups + 20 seconds rest + 1 set as many as possible
- Light weight - 4x12 reps front raises +20
- Light weight - 4x12 reps side raises +20
- Light weight - 4x12 reps shoulder press +20
- Light weight - 4x12 reps triceps drop +20
- Light weight - 4x12 reps basic squats ++20
- Light weight - 4x12 reps reverse flyes +20
- 10 minutes strong run @80-90% effort
- Walking lunges – with light weight, 4x12 reps +20
- Static lunges with weights 10x6 +20

Cool down
15 minutes light aerobic jog, followed by stretching
- Adductor stretch 4 x 20 +30
- Gluteal stretch 4x20 +30
- Hamstring stretch 4x20 +30

PM
- **Swimming** 60 minutes.

WEEK 3
MONDAY, WEDNESDAY AND FRIDAY

AM
- Warm up 8-10 minutes – starting with 3-4 minutes of mobility, then follow with 3-4 minutes of light aerobic activity.

Core set
- 10x90 seconds front plank +20
- 10x40 side plank +20 + scissors plank

Basic Plyometric set
- 8x8 Double leg jumps in a row +20
- 6x8 spin and squat (no weight) +20
- Light 10 minute jog
- 12x12 basic upward jumps - with 30-45 rest after each 8 jumps (use light weight).

Core, and dynamic power set
- Indo Twists (or without Indo Board) 14x30 seconds of the exercise then 60 seconds rest.
- 6x8 Spin and stick on BOSU +20

Strength and Endurance Set
- 8x12 press ups + 20 seconds rest + 1 set as many as possible
- Light weight - 6x12 reps front raises +20
- Light weight - 6x12 reps side raises +20
- Light weight - 6x12 reps shoulder press +20
- Light weight - 6x12 reps triceps drop +20
- Light weight - 6x12 reps basic squats +20
- Light weight - 6x12 reps reverse flyes +20
- 10 minutes strong run @80-90% effort
- Walking lunges – with light weight, 4x12 reps +20
- Static lunges with weights 10x6 +20

Cool down
15 minutes light aerobic jog, followed by stretching
- Adductor stretch 4 x 20 +30
- Gluteal stretch 4x20 +30
- Hamstring stretch 4x20 +30

PM
- **Swimming** 60 minutes.

WEEK 4
MONDAY, WEDNESDAY AND FRIDAY

AM
- Warm up 8-10 minutes – starting with 3-4 minutes of mobility, then follow with 3-4 minutes of light aerobic activity.

Core set
- 10x90 seconds front plank +20
- 10x40 seconds side plank +20 + scissors plank

Basic Plyometric set
- 8x8 Double leg jumps in a row +20
- 6x8 spin and squat (no weight) +20
- Light 10 minute jog
- 12x12 basic upward jumps – with 30-45 rest after each 8 jumps (use light weight)

Core, and dynamic power set
- Indo Twists (or without Indo Board) 14x 30 seconds of the exercise then 60 seconds rest.
- 6x8 Spin and stick on BOSU +20

Strength and Endurance Set
- 8x12 press ups + 20 seconds rest + 1 set as many as possible.
- Light weight - 6x12 reps front raises +20
- Light weight - 6x12 reps side raises +20
- Light weight - 6x12 reps shoulder press +20
- Light weight - 6x12 reps triceps drop +20
- Light weight - 6x12 reps basic squats +20
- Light weight - 6x12 reps reverse flyes +20
- 10 minutes strong run @80-90% effort
- Walking lunges – with light weight, 4x12 reps +20
- Static lunges with weights 10x6 +20

Cool down
15 minutes light aerobic jog, followed by stretching
- Adductor stretch 4x20 +30
- Gluteal stretch 4x20 +30
- Hamstring stretch 4x20 +30

PM
- **Swimming** 60 minutes.

WEEK 5
MONDAY, WEDNESDAY AND FRIDAY

AM
- Warm up 8-10 minutes – starting with 3-4 minutes of mobility, then follow with 3-4 minutes of light aerobic activity.

Core set
- 10x90 seconds front plank +20
- 10x40 seconds side plank +20 + scissors plank

Basic Plyometric set
- 8x8 Double leg jumps in a row +20
- 6x8 spin and squat+30 no weight + 10 press ups after each set (super set)
- Light 10 minute jog
- 12x12 basic upward jumps – with 30-45 rest after each 8 jumps (use light weight)

Core, and dynamic power set
- Indo Twists (or without Indo Board) 14x30 seconds of the exercise then 60 seconds rest.
- 8x8 Spin and stick on BOSU +20

Strength and Endurance Set
- 8x12 press ups + 20 seconds rest + 1 set as many as possible.
- Light weight - 8x16 reps front raises +20
- Light weight - 8x16 reps side raises +20
- Light weight - 8x16 reps shoulder press +20
- Light weight - 8x16 reps triceps drop +20
- Light weight - 8x16 reps basic squats +20
- Light weight - 8x16 reps reverse flyes +20
- 10 minutes strong run @80-90% effort
- Walking lunges – with light weight, 8x12 reps +20
- Static lunges with weights 10x6 +20

Cool down
15 minutes light aerobic jog, followed by stretching
- Adductor stretch 4 x 20 +30
- Gluteal stretch 4x20 +30
- Hamstring stretch 4x20 +30

PM
- **Swimming** 60 minutes.

WEEK 6
MONDAY, WEDNESDAY AND FRIDAY

AM

- Warm up 8-10 minutes – starting with 3-4 minutes of mobility, then follow with 3-4 minutes of light aerobic activity.

Core set
- 10x90 seconds front plank +20
- 10x40 seconds side plank +20 + scissors plank

Basic Plyometric set
- 8x8 Double leg jumps in a row +20
- 6x8 spin and squat + 30 no weight + 10 press ups after each set (super set)
- Light 10 minute jog
- 12x12 basic upward jumps – with 30-45 rest after each 8 jumps (use light weight)

Core, and dynamic power set
- Indo Twists (or without Indo Board) 14x30 seconds of the exercise then 60 seconds rest.
- 8x8 Spin and stick on BOSU +20

Strength and Endurance Set
- 8x12 press ups +20 + 1 set as many as possible.
- Light weight - 8x16 reps front raises +20
- Light weight - 8x16 reps side raises +20
- Light weight - 8x16 reps shoulder press +20
- Light weight - 8x16 reps triceps drop +20
- Light weight - 8x16 reps basic squats +20 + weight
- Light weight - 8x16 reps reverse flyes +20
- 10 minutes strong run @80-90% effort +5 minutes at 70%
- Walking lunges – with light weight, 8x12 reps +20
- Static lunges with weights 10x6 +20

Cool down
15 minutes light aerobic jog, followed by stretching
- Adductor stretch 4x20 +30
- Gluteal stretch 4x20 +30
- Hamstring stretch 4x20 +30

PM
- **Swimming** 60 minutes.

WEEK 7
MONDAY, WEDNESDAY AND FRIDAY

AM

- Warm up 8-10 minutes – starting with 3-4 minutes of mobility, then follow with 3-4 minutes of light aerobic activity.

Core set
- 10x90 seconds front plank +20
- 10x40 seconds side plank +20 + scissors plank

Basic Plyometric set
- 8x8 Double leg jumps in a row +20
- 6x8 spin and squat + 30 no weight + 10 press ups after each set (super set)
- Light 10 minute jog
- 12x12 basic upward jumps – with 30-45 rest after each 8 jumps (use light weight)

Core, and dynamic power set
- Indo Twists (or without Indo Board) 14x30 seconds of the exercise then 60 seconds rest.
- 8x8 Spin and stick on BOSU +20

Strength and Endurance Set
- 8x12 press ups + 20 seconds rest + 1 set as many as possible
- Light weight - 6x16 reps front raises +20
- Light weight - 6x16 reps side raises +20
- Light weight - 6x16 reps shoulder press +20
- Light weight - 6x16 reps triceps drop +20
- Light weight - 6x16 reps basic squats +20 + weight
- Light weight - 6x16 reps reverse flyes +20
- 10 minutes strong run @80-90% effort + 5 minutes at 70%
- Walking lunges – with light weight, 8x12 reps +20
- Static lunges with weights 10x6+20

Cool down
15 minutes light aerobic jog, followed by stretching
- Adductor stretch 4x20 +30
- Gluteal stretch 4x20 +30
- Hamstring stretch 4x20 +30

PM
- **Swimming** 60 minutes.

WEEK 8
MONDAY, WEDNESDAY AND FRIDAY

AM

- Warm up 8-10 minutes – starting with 3-4 minutes of mobility, then follow with 3-4 minutes of light aerobic activity.

Core set
- 10x90 seconds front plank +20
- 10x40 seconds side plank +20 + scissors plank

Basic Plyometric set
- 8x8 Double leg jumps in a row +20
- 6x8 spin and squat + 30 no weight + 10 press ups after each set (super set)
- Light 10 minute jog
- 12x12 basic upward jumps – with 30-45 rest after each 8 jumps (use light weight)

Core, and dynamic power set
- Indo Twists (or without Indo Board) 14x30 seconds of the exercise then 60 seconds rest.
- 8x8 Spin and stick on BOSU +20

Strength and Endurance Set
- 8x12 press ups + 20 seconds rest + 1 set as many as possible
- Light weight - 8x16 reps front raises +20
- Light weight - 8x16 reps side raises +20
- Light weight - 8x16 reps shoulder press +20
- Light weight - 8x16 reps triceps drop +20
- Light weight - 8x16 reps basic squats +20 + weight
- Light weight - 8x16 reps reverse flyes +20
- 10 minutes strong run @80-90% effort + 5 minutes at 70%
- Walking lunges – with light weight, 8x12 reps +20
- Static lunges with weights 10x6 +20

Cool down
15 minutes light aerobic jog, followed by stretching
- Adductor stretch 4 x 20 +30
- Gluteal stretch 4x20 +30
- Hamstring stretch 4x20 +30

PM
- **Swimming** 60 minutes.

WEEK 9
MONDAY, WEDNESDAY AND FRIDAY

AM

- Warm up 8-10 minutes – starting with 3-4 minutes of mobility, then follow with 3-4 minutes of light aerobic activity.

Core set
- 10x1.45 seconds front plank +20 + 10 squat thrusts (super set)
- 10x40 side plank +20 + scissors plank

Basic Plyometric set
- 10x8 Double leg jumps in a row +15
- 6x8 spin and squat + 30 no weight + 15 press ups after each set (super set)
- Light 10 minute jog
- 12x12 basic upward jumps – with 30-45 rest after each 8 jumps (use light weight)

Core, and dynamic power set
- Indo Twists (or without Indo Board) 14x30 seconds of the exercise then 60 seconds rest.
- 10x8 Spin and stick on BOSU +20
- 10 minutes strong run @80-90% effort

Strength and Endurance Set
- 8x12 press ups +20 + 1 set as many as possible
- Light weight - 8x16 reps front raises +20
- Light weight - 8x16 reps side raises +20
- Light weight - 8x16 reps shoulder press +20
- Light weight - 8x16 reps triceps drop +20
- Light weight - 8x16 reps basic squats +20 + weight
- Light weight - 8x16 reps reverse flyes +20
- 10 minutes strong run @80-90% effort + 5 minutes at 70%
- Walking lunges – with light weight, 8x12 reps +20
- Static lunges with weights 10x6 +20

Cool down
15 minutes light aerobic jog, followed by stretching
- Adductor stretch 4x20 +30
- Gluteal stretch 4x20 +30
- Hamstring stretch 4x20 +30

PM
- **Swimming** 60 minutes.

WEEK 10
MONDAY, WEDNESDAY AND FRIDAY

AM

- Warm up 8-10 minutes – starting with 3-4 minutes of mobility, then follow with 3-4 minutes of light aerobic activity.

Core set
- 10x1.45 seconds front plank +20 + 10 squat thrusts (super set)
- 10x40 side plank +20 + scissors plank

Basic Plyometric set
- 10x8 Double leg jumps in a row +15
- 6x8 spin and squat + 30 no weight + 15 press ups after each set (super set)
- Light 10 minute jog
- 12x12 basic upward jumps – with 30-45 rest after each 8 jumps (use light weight)

Core, and dynamic power set
- Indo Twists (or without Indo Board) 14x30 seconds of the exercise then 60 seconds rest
- 10x8 Spin and stick on BOSU +20
- 10 minutes strong run @80-90% effort

Strength and Endurance Set
- 8x12 press ups +20 + 1 set as many as possible
- Light weight - 8x16 reps front raises +20
- Light weight - 8x16 reps side raises +20
- Light weight - 8x16 reps shoulder press +20
- Light weight - 8x16 reps triceps drop +20
- Light weight - 8x16 reps basic squats +20 + weight
- Light weight - 8x16 reps reverse flyes +20
- 10 minutes strong run @80-90% effort- + 5 minutes at 70%
- Walking lunges – with light weight, 8x12 reps +20
- Static lunges with weights 10x6 +20

Cool down
15 minutes light aerobic jog, followed by stretching
- Adductor stretch 4x20 +30
- Gluteal stretch 4x20 +30
- Hamstring stretch 4x20 +30

PM
- **Swimming** 60 minutes.

WEEK 11
MONDAY, WEDNESDAY AND FRIDAY

AM

- Warm up 8-10 minutes – starting with 3-4 minutes of mobility, then follow with 3-4 minutes of light Aerobic activity.

Core set
- 10x1.45 seconds front plank +20 + 10 squat thrusts (super set)
- 10x40 side plank +20 + scissors plank

Basic Plyometric set
- 10x8 Double leg jumps in a row +15
- 6x10 spin and squat + 30 no weight + 15 press ups after each set (super set)
- Light 10 minute jog
- 14x12 basic upward jumps – with 30-45 rest after each 8 jumps(use light weight)

Core, and dynamic power set
- Indo Twists (or without Indo Board) 14x30 seconds of the exercise then 60 seconds rest
- 10x8 Spin and stick on BOSU +20
- 10 minutes strong run @80-90% effort

Strength and Endurance Set
- 8x12 press ups +20 + 1 set as many as possible
- Light weight - 8x16 reps front raises +20
- Light weight - 8x16 reps side raises +20
- Light weight - 8x16 reps shoulder press +20
- Light weight - 8x16 reps triceps drop +20
- Light weight - 8x16 reps basic squats +20 + weight
- Light weight - 8x16 reps reverse flyes +20
- 10 minutes strong run @80-90% effort + 5 minutes at 70%
- Walking lunges – with light weight, 8x12 reps +20
- Static lunges with weights 10x6 +20

Cool down
15 minutes light aerobic jog, followed by stretching
- Adductor stretch 4x20 +30
- Gluteal stretch 4x20 +30
- Hamstring stretch 4x20 +30

PM
- **Swimming** 60 minutes.

WEEK 12
MONDAY, WEDNESDAY AND FRIDAY

AM

- Warm up 8-10 minutes – starting with 3-4 minutes of mobility, then follow with 3-4 minutes of light aerobic activity.

Core set
- 10x1.45 seconds front plank +20 + 10 squat thrusts (super set)
- 10x40 side plank +20 + scissors plank

Basic Plyometric set
- 10x8 Double leg jumps in a row +15
- 6x8 spin and squat + 30 no weight + 15 press ups after each set (super set)
- Light 10 minute jog
- 16x12 basic upward jumps – with 30-45 rest after each 8 jumps (use light weight)

Core, and dynamic power set
- Indo Twists (or without Indo Board) 16x 30 seconds of the exercise then 60 seconds rest
- 14x8 Spin and stick on BOSU +20
- 10 minutes strong run @80-90% effort + 5 mins at 70%

Strength and Endurance Set
- 8x12 press ups +20 + 1 set as many as possible
- Light weight - 8x16 reps front raises +20
- Light weight - 8x16 reps side raises +20
- Light weight - 8x16 reps shoulder press +20
- Light weight - 8x16 reps triceps drop +20
- Light weight - 8x16 reps basic squats +20 + weight
- Light weight - 8x16 reps reverse flyes +20
- 10 minutes strong run @80-90% effort + 5 minutes at 70%
- Walking lunges – with light weight, 8x12 reps +20
- Static lunges with weights 10x6 +20

Cool down
15 minutes light aerobic jog, followed by stretching
- Adductor stretch 4x20 +30
- Gluteal stretch 4x20 +30
- Hamstring stretch 4x20 +30

PM
- **Swimming** 60 minutes.

WEEK 13
MONDAY, WEDNESDAY AND FRIDAY

AM

- Warm up 8-10 minutes – starting with 3-4 minutes of mobility, then follow with 3-4 minutes of light aerobic activity.

Core set
- 10x 2.00 seconds front plank +20 + 15 squat thrusts (super set)
- 10x40 side plank +20 + scissors plank

Basic Plyometric set
- 16x8 Double leg jumps in a row +15
- 6x8 spin and squat+30no weight + 15 press ups after each set (super set)
- Light 10 minute jog
- 16x12 basic upward jumps – with 30-45 rest after each 8 jumps (use light weight)

Core, and dynamic power set
- Indo Twists (or without Indo Board) 16x 40 seconds of the exercise then 60 seconds rest
- 14x8 Spin and stick on BOSU +20
- 10 minutes strong run @80-90% effort + 5 mins at 70%+

Strength and Endurance Set
- 16x12 press ups +20 + 1 set as many as possible
- Light weight - 8x16 reps front raises +20
- Light weight - 8x16 reps side raises +20
- Light weight - 8x16 reps shoulder press +20
- Light weight - 8x16 reps triceps drop +20
- Light weight - 8x16 reps basic squats +20 + weight
- Light weight - 8x16 reps reverse flyes +20
- 10 minutes strong run @80-90% effort + 5 minutes at 70%
- Walking lunges – with light weight, 8x12 reps +20
- Static lunges with weights 10x6 +20
- 5 minute run @ 95-100%

Cool down
15 minutes light aerobic jog, followed by stretching
- Adductor stretch 4x20 +30
- Gluteal Stretch 4x20 +30
- Hamstring stretch 4x20 +30

PM
- **Swimming** 60 minutes.

WEEK 14
MONDAY, WEDNESDAY AND FRIDAY

AM

- Warm up 8-10 minutes – starting with 3-4 minutes of mobility, then follow with 3-4 minutes of light aerobic activity.

Core set
- 10x2.00 seconds front plank +20 + 10 squat thrusts (super set)
- 10x40 side plank +20 + scissors plank

Basic Plyometric set
- 16x8 Double leg jumps in a row +15
- 6x8 spin and squat + 30 no weight + 15 press ups after each set (super set)
- Light 10 minute jog
- 16x16 basic upward jumps – with 30-45 rest after each 8 jumps (use light weight)

Core, and dynamic power set
- Indo Twists (or without Indo Board) 16x 30 seconds of the exercise then 60 seconds rest
- 14x8 Spin and stick on BOSU +20
- 10 minutes strong run @80-90% effort + 5 mins at 70%+

Strength and Endurance Set
- 15x12 press ups +20 + 1 set as many as possible
- Light weight - 8x16 reps front raises +20
- Light weight - 8x16 reps side raises +20
- Light weight - 8x16 reps shoulder press +20
- Light weight - 8x16 reps triceps drop +20
- Light weight - 8x16 reps basic squats +20 + weight
- Light weight - 8x16 reps reverse flyes +20
- 10 minutes strong run @80-90% effort + 5 minutes at 70%
- Walking lunges – with light weight, 8x12 reps +20
- Static lunges with weights 10x6 +20
- 5 minute run @ 95-100%

Cool down
15 minutes light aerobic jog, followed by stretching
- Adductor stretch 4 x 20 +30
- Gluteal stretch 4x20 +30
- Hamstring stretch 4x20 +30

PM
- **Swimming** 60 minutes.

WEEK 15
MONDAY, WEDNESDAY AND FRIDAY

AM
- Warm up 8-10 minutes – starting with 3-4 minutes of mobility, then follow with 3-4 minutes of light aerobic activity.

Core set
- 10x2.00 seconds front plank +20 + 10 squat thrusts (super set)
- 10x40 seconds side plank +20 + scissors plank

Basic Plyometric set
- 16x 8 Double leg jumps in a row +15
- 6x8 spin and squat + 30 no weight + 15 press ups after each set (super set)
- Light 10 minute jog
- 16x16 basic upward jumps – with 30-45 rest after each 8 jumps (use light weight)

Core, and dynamic power set
- Indo Twists (or without Indo Board) 16x40 seconds of the exercise then 60 seconds rest
- 14x8 Spin and stick on BOSU +20
- 10 minutes strong run @80-90% effort + 5 mins at 70%+

Strength and Endurance Set
- 8x12press ups +20 + 1 set as many as possible
- Light weight - 8x16 reps front raises +20
- Light weight - 8x16 reps side raises ++20
- Light weight - 8x16 reps shoulder press +20
- Light weight - 8x16 reps triceps drop +20
- Light weight - 8x16 reps basic squats +20+ weight
- Light weight - 8x16 reps reverse flyes +20
- 10 minutes strong run @80-90% effort + 5 minutes at 70%
- Walking lunges – with light weight, 8x12 reps +20
- Static lunges with weights 10x6 +20
- 5 minute run @ 95-100%

Cool down
15 minutes light aerobic jog, followed by stretching
- Adductor stretch 4x20 +30
- Gluteal stretch 4x20 +30
- Hamstring stretch 4x20 +30

PM
- **Swimming** 60 minutes.

WEEK 16
MONDAY, WEDNESDAY AND FRIDAY

AM
- Warm up 8-10 minutes – starting with 3-4 minutes of mobility, then follow with 3-4 minutes of light aerobic activity.

Core set
- 10x2.00 seconds front plank +20 + 10 squat thrusts (super set)
- 10x40 seconds side plank +20 + scissors plank

Basic Plyometric set
- 10x8 Double leg jumps in a row +15
- 12x8 spin and squat + 30 no weight + 15 press ups after each set (super set)
- Light 10 minute jog
- 16x18 basic upward jumps – with 30-45 rest after each 8 jumps (use light weight)

Core, and dynamic power set
- Indo Twists (or without Indo Board) 16x 30 seconds of the exercise then 60 seconds rest
- 14x15 Spin and stick on BOSU +20
- 10 minutes strong run @80-90% effort + 5 mins at 70%+

Strength and Endurance Set
- 8x16 press ups +20 + 1 set as many as possible
- Light weight - 8x18 reps front raises +20
- Light weight - 8x18 reps side raises +20
- Light weight - 8x18 reps shoulder press +20
- Light weight - 8x18 reps triceps drop +20
- Light weight - 8x18 reps basic squats +20 + weight
- Light weight - 8x18 reps reverse flyes +20
- 10 minutes strong run @80-90% effort + 5 minutes at 70%
- Walking lunges – with light weight, 8x15 reps +20
- Static lunges with weights 10x8 +20
- 5 minute run @ 95-100%

Cool down
15 minutes light aerobic jog, followed by stretching
- Adductor stretch 4x20 +30
- Gluteal stretch 4x20 +30
- Hamstring stretch 4x20 +30

PM
- **Swimming** 60 minutes.

CONCLUSION

NOW YOU'VE COMPLETED THE BASIC, INTERMEDIATE AND ADVANCED TRAINING PLANS, MAINTENANCE IS NOW KEY, FOLLOW A GOOD PROGRAMME AND KEEP IT MAINTAINED!

Land Training will become part of your surfing programme of development , you will feel it in the water, and in your day to day activity's.

Add new and different exercises to your work out monthly.

Stay focused keep your training up weekly for best results!

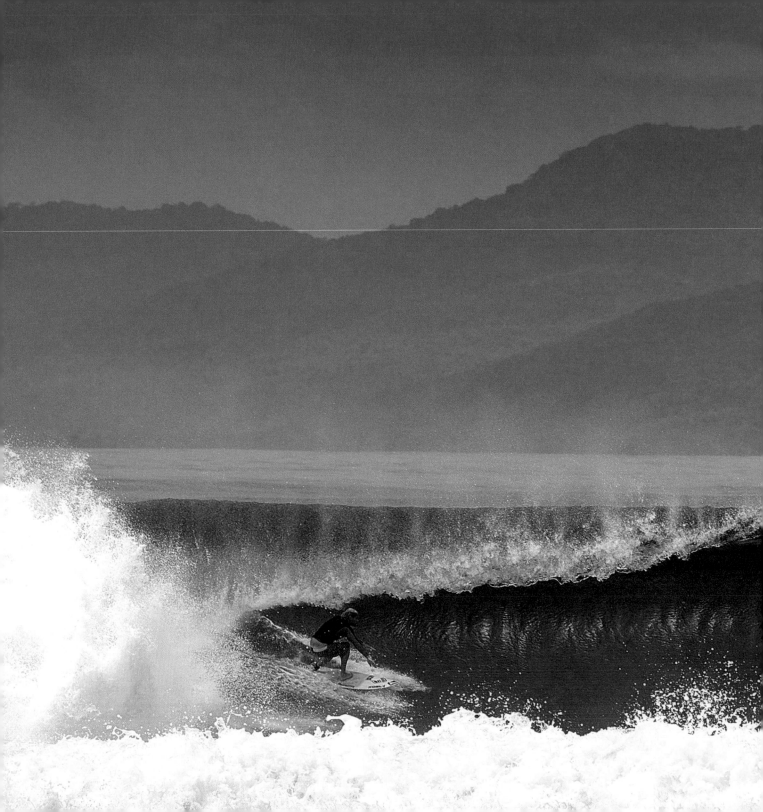

FINAL TIPS

Whichever way you go with your training aim for regular sessions.

PROGRESSION

Progression is key, exercises that mimic a surfing movement will always be best.

DIVERSITY

Diversify and change your programme subject to needs and requirements.

SURF MORE

Always warm up, always cool down, surf longer, stay fitter and catch more waves!

ABOUT US

LEE STANBURY

Surfer Lee Stanbury has 25 years' experience in the leisure and fitness industry. He is an experienced head swim coach and personal trainer. He's also MD and Owner of Big Blue Sports Distribution, Fit4swimming.co.uk and Fit2surf.com. In his spare time (when he's not writing for publications such as Swimming Times, Carve Surfing Magazine and SurfGirl) Lee found the time to invent Powerstroke Cords as an aid to improve paddling strength. Never one to let the grass grow under his feet he is now a 'worn out dad' with three children under four years old – and still sometimes finds time to pull into the occasional barrel at his local beach.

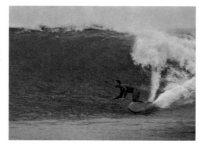

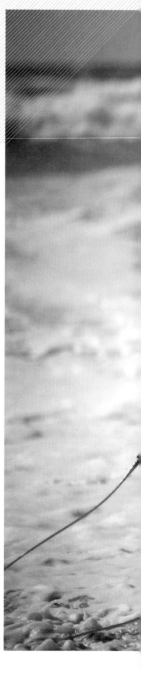

LEE BARTLETT

Lee Bartlett was raised in the UK surfing capital Newquay. Lee embarked on a competitive surf career in his early years and has 20 British and English national titles across there divisions. These days Lee is the head shaper for Toy Factory Surfboards and an in demand contest commentator. He says his ambition is to "stay fit, keep surfing and have fun".

SHARPY

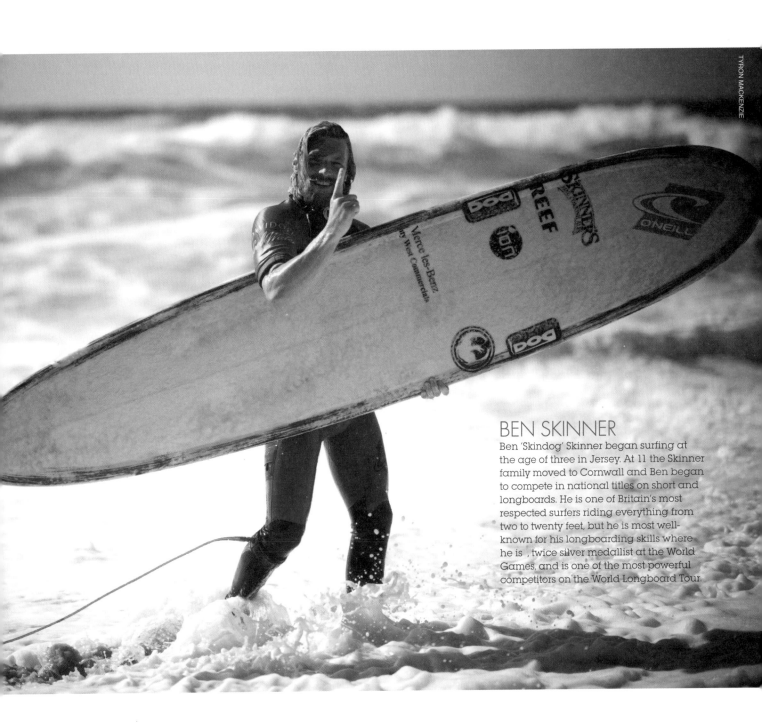

BEN SKINNER

Ben 'Skindog' Skinner began surfing at the age of three in Jersey. At 11 the Skinner family moved to Cornwall and Ben began to compete in national titles on short and longboards. He is one of Britain's most respected surfers riding everything from two to twenty feet, but he is most well-known for his longboarding skills where he is , twice silver medallist at the World Games, and is one of the most powerful competitors on the World Longboard Tour.

INDEX

FURTHER READING

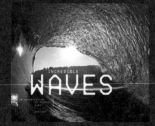

INCREDIBLE WAVES
By Chris Power
ISBN 978-0-9567893-3-4

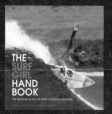

THE SURF GIRL HANDBOOK
By Louise Searle
ISBN 978-0-9523646-1-0

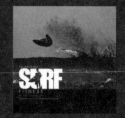

**THE COMPLETE GUIDE
TO SURF FITNESS**
By Lee Stanbury
ISBN 978-0-9523646-6-5

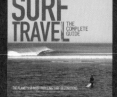

**SURF TRAVEL –
THE COMPLETE GUIDE**
Edited by Chris Power
ISBN 978-0-9523646-9-6

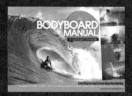

**THE BODYBOARD
MANUAL**
Edited by Rob Barber
ISBN 978-0-9567893-5-8

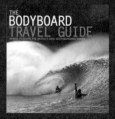

**THE BODYBOARD TRAVEL
GUIDE**
By Owen Pye with Rob
Barber and Mike Searle
ISBN 978-0-9567893-0-3

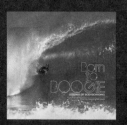

**BORN TO BOOGIE –
LEGENDS OF
BODYBOARDING**
by Owen Pye
ISBN 978-0-9567893-2-7

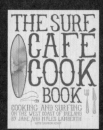

**THE SURF CAFÉ
COOKBOOK**
By Jane and Myles Lamberth
with Shannon Denny
ISBN 978-0-9567893-1-0

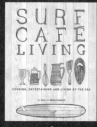

SURF CAFÉ LIVING
By Jane and Myles
Lamberth
ISBN 978-0-9567893-6-5

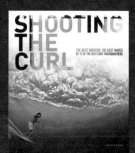

SHOOTING THE CURL
By Chris Power
ISBN 978-0-9523646-8-9

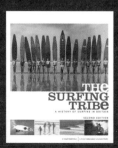

**THE SURFING TRIBE:
A HISTORY OF SURFING
IN BRITAIN**
By Roger Mansfield
ISBN 978-0-9523646-0-3

MAGAZINES

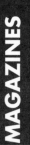

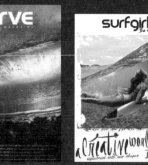

**CARVE SURFING
MAGAZINE**

**SURFGIRL
MAGAZINE**